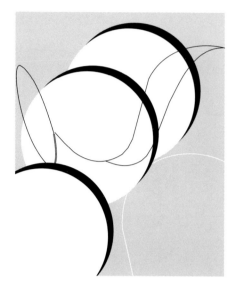

GLENN T. CLARK, DDS, MS
Associate Dean of Research
Professor and Director
UCLA Dental Research Institute
Center for Health Sciences
Los Angeles, CA

BRUCE SANDERS, DDS
Adjunct Professor, Section of
Oral and Maxillofacial Surgery
UCLA School of Dentistry
Center for Health Sciences
Los Angeles, CA
Senior Staff, Saint John's
Hospital and Health Center,
Santa Monica, CA

**CHARLES N. BERTOLAMI, DDS,
DMedSc**
Professor and Chairman, Section of
Oral and Maxillofacial Surgery
UCLA School of Dentistry
Center for Health Sciences
Los Angeles, CA

Advances in Diagnostic and Surgical Arthroscopy of the Temporomandibular Joint

W.B. SAUNDERS COMPANY
Harcourt Brace Jovanovich, Inc.
Philadelphia London Toronto Montreal Sydney Tokyo

W.B. SAUNDERS COMPANY
Harcourt Brace Jovanovich, Inc.

The Curtis Center
Independence Square West
Philadelphia, Pennsylvania 19106

Library of Congress Cataloging-in-Publication Data

Advances in diagnostic and surgical arthroscopy of the
temporomandibular joint / [edited by] Glenn T. Clark, Bruce Sanders,
Charles N. Bertolami.

p.   cm.

Includes bibliographical references and index.

ISBN 0-7216-6591-8

1. Temporomandibular joint—Diseases—Diagnosis.
   2. Temporomandibular joint—Surgery.   3. Arthroscopy.
   4. Temporomandibular Joint—surgery.   5. Temporomandibular
Joint Diseases—diagnosis.

[DNLM: 1. Arthroscopy. WU 140 M689]

RK470.M63   1993

617.5'22—dc20
DNLM/DLC   92-11625

**ADVANCES IN DIAGNOSTIC AND SURGICAL ARTHROSCOPY
OF THE TEMPOROMANDIBULAR JOINT**   ISBN 0–7216–6591–8

Printed in the United States of America.

Last digit is the print number: 9   8   7   6   5   4   3   2   1

CONTRIBUTORS

CHARLES N. BERTOLAMI, D.D.S., D.Med.Sc.

Professor and Chairman, Section of Oral and Maxillofacial Surgery, UCLA School of Dentistry, Center for Health Sciences, Los Angeles, California

CAROL A. BIBB, Ph.D., D.D.S.

Adjunct Associate Professor, Section of Orofacial Pain & Occlusion, UCLA School of Dentistry, Los Angeles, California

  The Histologic Basis and Clinical Implications for Temporomandibular Joint Adaptation

LAMBERT G.M. de BONT, D.D.S., Ph.D.

Associate Professor, University of Groningen; Staff Member, Department of Oral and Maxillofacial Surgery, University Hospital, Groningen, The Netherlands

  Terminology for Normal Findings

JON BRADRICK, D.D.S.

Assistant Professor of Surgery, College of Medicine, Case Western Reserve University; Staff Oral and Maxillofacial Surgeon, Department of Surgery, Metro-Health Medical Center, Cleveland, Ohio

  Arthroscopic Laser Procedures; Development of the Canine Model for Investigative Temporomandibular Joint Arthroscopy

RALPH D. BUONCRISTIANI, D.D.S.

Visiting Lecturer, Department of Oral and Maxillofacial Surgery, and Clinical Professor, Continuing Education in Dentistry, UCLA School of Dentistry, Los Angeles, California; Staff Member, St. John's Hospital and Health Center, and Santa Monica Hospital Medi-cal Center, Santa Monica, California; UCLA Medical Center, Los Angeles, California

  A 5-Year Experience with Arthroscopic Lysis and Lavage for the Treatment of Painful Temporomandibular Joint Hypomobility; Temporomandibular Joint Arthroscopic Photography and Documentation Techniques

BRUCE B. CHISHOLM, D.D.S.

Resident, Oral and Maxillofacial Surgery Graduate Training Program, University of Missouri—Kansas City School of Dentistry, Kansas City, Missouri

  Effectiveness of Arthroscopy: A Retrospective Study

GLENN T. CLARK, D.D.S., M.S.

Associate Dean of Research, Professor and Director, UCLA Dental Research Institute, Center for Health Sciences, Los Angeles, California

  Arthroscopic Treatment of the Human Temporomandibular Joint; Sodium Hyaluronate Injections in Synovial Joints

JOHN F. DISTEFANO, D.D.S.

Associate Clinical Professor, Department of Oral and Maxillofacial Surgery, Case Western Reserve University School of Dentistry; Active Staff Member, University Hospitals of Cleveland, Cleveland, Ohio

  Arthroscopic Evaluation of Patients with Temporary Silastic Implants

BRETT L. FERGUSON, D.D.S.

Associate Professor, Schools of Medicine and Dentistry, and Director, Outpatient Clinics, University of Missouri—Kansas City; Staff Member, Truman Medi-

cal Center; Children's Mercy Hospital; Trinity Lutheran Hospital, Kansas City, Missouri
> Effectiveness of Arthroscopy: A Retrospective Study

JEROLD S. GOLDBERG, D.D.S.

Professor and Chairman, Department of Oral and Maxillofacial Surgery, Case Western Reserve University; Director of Oral and Maxillofacial Surgery, University Hospitals of Cleveland, Cleveland, Ohio
> Arthroscopic Evaluation of Patients with Temporary Silastic Implants; Synovial Fluid Pressure

A. THOMAS INDRESANO, D.M.D.

Associate Professor of Oral and Maxillofacial Surgery, College of Medicine, Case Western Reserve University; Director, Oral and Maxillofacial Surgery, MetroHealth Medical Center, Cleveland, Ohio
> Arthroscopic Laser Procedures; Development of the Canine Model for Investigative Temporomandibular Joint Arthroscopy

RONALD M. KAMINISHI, D.D.S.

Clinical Professor, University of Southern California School of Dentistry, Bellflower, California; Assistant Professor, Loma Linda University School of Dentistry and School of Medicine, Loma Linda, California; Assistant Clinical Professor, University of California, Irvine, Medical Center, Irvine, California; Active Staff Member, Long Beach Memorial Medical Center, Long Beach, California
> Intracapsular Fibrosis Related to Pain and Dysfunction

TOSHIROU KONDOH, D.M.D., Ph.D.

Assistant Professor, Department of Oral and Maxillofacial Surgery, School of Dentistry, Tsurumi University; Director, Department of Oral and Maxillofacial Surgery, Yokohama Rosai Hospital, Yokohama, Japan
> Arthroscopic Traction Suturing: Treatment of Internal Derangement by Arthroscopic Repositioning and Suturing of the Disk

CHANGRUI LIU, D.D.S.

Research Associate, Dental Research Institute, UCLA School of Dentistry, Los Angeles, California
> Arthroscopic Treatment of the Human Temporomandibular Joint; Sodium Hyaluronate Injections in Synovial Joints

R. G. MERRILL, D.D.S., M.Sc.D.

Professor and Chairman, Department of Oral and Maxillofacial Surgery, Oregon Health Sciences University; Active Staff Member, Oregon Health Sciences University Hospital; Active Staff Member, Holladay Park Medical Center, Portland, Oregon
> Arthroscopic Temporomandibular Joint Lysis, Lavage, and Manipulation and Chemical Sclerotherapy for Painful Hypermobility and Recurrent Mandibular Dislocation

LARRY J. MOORE, D.D.S., M.S.

Lecturer, Department of Oral Pathology, UCLA School of Dentistry, Los Angeles, California; Chairman, Oral and Maxillofacial Surgery, Long Beach Memorial Medical Center, Long Beach, California
> Arthroscopic Surgery for the Treatment of Restrictive Temporomandibular Joint Disease: A Prospective Longitudinal Study

EDWARD L. MOSBY, D.D.S., F.A.C.D.

Professor, Oral and Maxillofacial Surgery, and Associate Director, Oral and Maxillofacial Surgery Graduate Training Program, Schools of Dentistry and Medicine, University of Missouri—Kansas City; Associate Chairman, Department of Dentistry, Truman Medical Center, Kansas City, Missouri
> Effectiveness of Arthroscopy: A Retrospective Study

JEFFREY J. MOSES, D.D.S.

Adjunct Assistant Professor, UCLA School of Dentistry, Los Angeles, California; Medical Director, Pacific Clinical Research Foundation, Encinitas, California; Associate Clinical Professor, Department of Oral and Maxillofacial Surgery, Loma Linda University, Loma Linda, California; Medical Staff Member, Tri-City Medical Center, Scripps Memorial Hospital, and Children's Hospital and Health Center, San Diego, California
> Temporomandibular Joint Arthroscopic Surgery: The Endaural Approach, Lateral Eminence Release, Capsular Stretch, and Articular Eminoplasty—Rationale and Technique

KEN-ICHIRO MURAKAMI, D.D.S., Ph.D.

Assistant Professor and Associate Head, Department of Oral and Maxillofacial Surgery, Faculty of Medicine, Kyoto University Hospital, Kyoto, Japan
> Intraarticular Adhesions of the Temporomandibular Joint: Arthroscopic Views and Clinical Perspectives

MASATOSHI OHNISHI, D.D.S., Ph.D.

Professor and Chairman, Department of Oral and Maxillofacial Surgery, Yamanashi Medical College, Yamanashi, Japan
> Arthroscopic Laser Surgery and Suturing for Temporomandibular Joint Disorders

BRADLEY T. PORTER, D.D.S., M.S.

Clinical Instructor, Meriter-Park Dental Clinic; Staff Member, Meriter-Park Hospital; Meriter-Capitol Hospital; St. Mary's Hospital Medical Center, Madison, Wisconsin

A Retrospective Study Comparing Arthroscopic Surgery with Arthrotomy and Disk Repositioning

ANDREW G. PULLINGER, D.D.S., M.Sc.

Associate Professor; Director, Postdoctoral Program in Orofacial Pain and Dysfunction; and Codirector, Pain Management Center, UCLA School of Dentistry, Los Angeles, California

The Histologic Basis and Clinical Implications for Temporomandibular Joint Adaptation

BRUCE SANDERS, D.D.S.

Adjunct Professor, Section of Oral and Maxillofacial Surgery, UCLA School of Dentistry, Center for Health Sciences, Los Angeles, California; Senior Staff, Saint John's Hospital and Health Center, Santa Monica, California

A 5-Year Experience with Arthroscopic Lysis and Lavage for the Treatment of Painful Temporomandibular Joint Hypomobility

NATSUKI SEGAMI, D.D.S., Ph.D.

Assistant Professor, Department of Oral and Maxillofacial Surgery, Faculty of Medicine, Kyoto University Hospital, Kyoto, Japan

Intraarticular Adhesions of the Temporomandibular Joint: Arthroscopic Views and Clinical Perspectives

BOUDEWIJN STEGENGA, D.M.D., Ph.D.

Research Associate, Department of Oral and Maxillofacial Surgery, University Hospital, Groningen, The Netherlands

Terminology for Normal Findings

DAVID A. SWANN, Ph.D.

Consultant, Department of Surgery, Massachusetts General Hospital, and Harvard Medical School, Boston, Massachusetts

The Structure and Function of Sodium Hyaluronate and Its Use as a Biomaterial to Treat Temporomandibular Joint Dysfunction

DANIEL C. TOPPER, D.D.S.

Previous Surgical Fellow at Pacific Clinical Research Foundation, Encinitas, California; Private Practice, Lakewood, Colorado

Temporomandibular Joint Arthroscopic Surgery: The Endaural Approach, Lateral Eminence Release, Capsular Stretch, and Articular Eminoplasty—Rationale and Technique

DEBORAH L. ZEITLER, D.D.S., M.S.

Associate Professor and Director, Oral and Maxillofacial Surgery Residency Program, University of Iowa; Staff Member, Department of Hospital Dentistry, Division of Oral and Maxillofacial Surgery, University of Iowa Hospitals and Clinics; Department of Dental Services, Department of Veterans Affairs Medical Center, Iowa City, Iowa

A Retrospective Study Comparing Arthroscopic Surgery with Arthrotomy and Disk Repositioning

PREFACE

The introduction of arthroscopy as a modality for the management of temporomandibular joint (TMJ) disorders has completely changed surgical goals. Today, TMJ surgery offers an opportunity for true rehabilitation. Specific TMJ function disorders that can benefit substantially, if not completely, from arthroscopic intervention can now be identified. The proceedings of our first symposium, *Diagnostic and Surgical Arthroscopy of the Temporomandibular Joint* (W. B. Saunders Co., 1988) introduced and documented the efficiency of TMJ arthroscopic surgery. This work proposed a nomenclature for recording arthroscopically visualized joint surface anatomy and presented the basic surgical approaches and techniques for the arthroscopic treatment of the acutely restricted joint. It proved to be of great interest to those involved in oral and maxillofacial surgery and the clinical management of TMJ disorders.

The proceedings from our second symposium, which are published in the present volume, represent a significant advance over the earlier work. The latest technical improvements in the imaging and recording of joint tissues are accurately and dynamically presented. Furthermore, improved understanding of joint tissue surface interfaces and advances in articular lubrication are presented in the chapters dealing with sodium hyaluronate. The remainder of the book is divided into sections addressing the diagnosis and treatment of TMJ disorders as well as technology and research in the management of TMJ pathology. Speakers from around the world participated in the symposium. Only by attempting a rational scientific review of the work being done in this field can we hope to understand and gain a broad-based perspective on this topic.

One area of controversy involves to what extent arthroscopic joint therapy can be applied in TMJ pathology. Specifically, for which problems (other than acute pathology, closed-lock, and chronic fibrous adhesions) does arthroscopic surgery offer a reasonable solution? New techniques for altering disk position using lasers, suturing, and cautery are presented. Animal models, synovial fluid pressure studies, and related topics are also discussed.

The editors would like to acknowledge the contributions of individuals, without whom neither the symposium nor this book would have been possible. First, we would like to thank the UCLA Continuing Education Department for its fine efforts and logistic support in conducting the symposium and for making it an enjoyable scientific meeting. In particular, Mr. Michael Vandiver and Dr. Ina Zive were instrumental in planning the symposium. Second, we wish to acknowledge the assistance of Dr. Robert Delcanho, who participated in much of the editing of the contributed materials. Also, we would like to thank the fine staff at W. B. Saunders Company, which has compiled these materials into an organized and comprehensive text. Lastly, and most important, the editors would like to thank all of the patients on whom our experience is based. Without them and their willingness to entrust us with their care, we would not have been able to learn as much about this area as we have. We hope this book will be valuable both to practitioners and to their patients.

GLENN T. CLARK
BRUCE SANDERS, AND
CHARLES N. BERTOLAMI,
Editors

CONTENTS

PART 1

Diagnosis

One

Terminology for Normal Findings

LAMBERT G.M. DE BONT, D.D.S., PH.D.
BOUDEWIJN STEGENGA, D.D.S., PH.D.

Using the term *normal* as an adjunct to *findings* suggests that there is an accepted standard for the findings obtained during arthroscopy of a temporomandibular joint (TMJ). A collection of randomly selected mandibles shows an enormous variation in shape and size of the condylar head. Standards for what is normal usually include such a range of *normal variation*, just like the area beneath the curve of a normal distribution reflects the normal variation of a biologic characteristic. Our judgments on morphology are based on these standards. For example, if only a midsagittal section of a normal-looking joint (i.e., without any pathology in that plane) is observed, we assume that the other parts will be normal as well. During arthroscopy, we are also dealing with a normal variation, especially in anatomy and in surface characteristics.

From 3-dimensional reconstructions from TMJ autopsy specimens a more realistic impression about TMJ morphology is obtained. Articular disks seem to have a normal variation in shape, size, and position. The condyle-disk relationship may frequently look quite normal although the disk has an unconventional form. Conversely, the condyle-disk relationship may be disturbed while the disk has a normal biconcave form. Again, the relevant questions are, what belongs to the normal variation and what is abnormal, and are we able to differentiate abnormality from normality during arthroscopy of the TMJ?

During arthroscopy, we also are dealing with a normal variation in surface characteristics. On inspection we should realize that the TMJ is a synovial joint, the basic elements of which are articular cartilage, the synovial membrane, and synovial fluid. This implies that while looking at the articular surfaces we have to

know what is going on within the articular tissues. The articular cartilage of the TMJ is composed of different layers or zones, and within each zone a specific architecture of the network is created by the collagen fibrils.[1] The collagen fibrils are intertwined proteoglycans, which consist of a protein core with numerous chains of keratan sulfate and chondroitin sulfate connected to a hyaluronic acid chain, thus creating large molecules. These proteoglycan aggregates are highly hydrophilic and form a swelling gel. In this way, the proteoglycans keep the collagen fibrils under constant tension and the articular cartilage acquires its physical properties. Although its articular cartilage consists of fibrocartilage instead of hyaline cartilage, the TMJ obeys the same laws as other synovial joints. The synovial fluid secreted by the synovial membrane is essential for joint lubrication and for sufficient nutrition of the cartilage cells, which occurs by diffusion from the synovial fluid.

When joint loading exceeds the adaptive capacity of the articular cartilage, degenerative changes of the cartilage result. Aging will also affect the joint structures and, consequently, the adaptive capacity of the joint. Age-related changes of articular cartilage take place in the collagen fibrils, the proteoglycans, and affect their interrelationship. So, when we observe degenerative changes, we should wonder whether they reflect real pathology or not. When there is pathology, and not simply an age-related change, we are talking about osteoarthrosis.

In our proposed classification of TMJ disorders, noninflammatory disorders are distinguished from inflammatory disorders.[2] Common noninflammatory TMJ disorders include osteoarthrosis, internal derangement, luxation, and subluxation. Frequently, inflammatory ar-

3

ticular disorders, like synovitis and capsulitis, are a secondary result of noninflammatory disorders.

Throughout life, the TMJ articular cartilage and the underlying bone display shifting equilibria between form and function by tissue remodeling, just as do the other joints in the body. Increased loading may stimulate remodeling, involving increased synthesis of proteoglycans and collagen fibrils. An overloading may disturb the equilibrium between form and function and give rise to tissue breakdown. In our osteoarthrosis concept, different conditions of the articular cartilage are described, from a normal variation to initial degenerative changes, possibly progressing to advanced changes, and finally to cartilage destruction.[3] In addition, we describe three stages of osteoarthrosis: an initial stage, an intermediate stage, and a terminal stage. In the initial stage signs and symptoms usually are absent. The clinical stages, from reducible disk displacement to permanent disk displacement that eventually progresses to a residual osteoarthrosis, are also included in our TMJ osteoarthrosis concept.

In the initial stage of osteoarthrosis, swelling and softening of the articular cartilage, resulting from an increased volume of the proteoglycan-water gel, is observed. Since no elements in the cartilage other than collagen have tensile strength, collagen fibril fragmentation is the most acceptable explanation for the increased hydration of the articular cartilage. In addition, proteoglycan depletion and the clustering of chondrocytes are observed in the early stage of osteoarthrosis.[4,5] The cells proliferate and become very active in an attempt to repair the lost matrix. The term "chondromalacia" is used rather loosely by medical professionals to describe a clinically distinct posttraumatic softening of the articular cartilage of the patella in young persons. Nowadays, it is also applied to the TMJ. The anatomic lesions due to chondromalacia are microscopically indistinguishable from those of early osteoarthrosis.

If we may compare chondromalacia of the patella with chondromalacia of the TMJ, we may also compare the arthroscopic findings of the patella with those of the TMJ. Although patellar articular surface alterations are not necessarily symptom-producing, a high incidence of such changes are described by Johnson.[6] The cartilage in areas with bacon-strip changes and bubble defects (also called blister formation) is swollen owing to the increased uptake of water, caused by a focal disruption of the collagen network and increased hydration, subsequent swelling of the proteoglycans, and fragmentation of the articular cartilage. These changes are also frequently present in the TMJ, especially in the lateral portion. Thus, in TMJ chondromalacia the integrity of the tissues is affected, but the condition

may be clinically bland. Although the articular surface may look normal during arthroscopic inspection of the joint structures, palpation with a blunt or hooked probe provides information about the softness of the tissue and enables the examination of small defects. Such instruments give us an idea of the magnification with which we examine these defects.

The initial degenerative changes not only are present at the articular surface and in the superficial layers of the articular zone but also exist in the deeper layers of the articular cartilage (splitting of the cartilage) and in the subchondral bone (fibrosis of the marrow spaces).[5] However, during arthroscopic inspection we are able to judge surface characteristics and to partly examine the articular cartilage, but we are certainly not able to make statements about the deeper layers of the articular cartilage and about the subchondral bone. Consequently, arthroscopy is limited to a part of the evaluation process. In addition, some characteristics, such as fibrous adhesions, are easily interpretable, but what about petechiae at the roof of the fossa or vascular patterns at the medial capsular wall of the joint? Future research on joint pathology should explain what is going on in the TMJ.

SUMMARY

In order to distinguish abnormal from normal findings during arthroscopy, the characteristics of TMJ pathology must be distinguished from those of a healthy TMJ. TMJ pathology must be considered as synovial joint pathology, and for the proper use of terms, TMJ terminology should, therefore, be synovial joint terminology.

REFERENCES

1. de Bont, LGM; Boering, G; Havinga, P; Liem, RSB. Spatial arrangement of collagen fibrils in the articular cartilage of the mandibular condyle: A light microscopic and scanning electron microscopic study. J Oral Maxillofac Surg (1984), 42:306–313.
2. Stegenga, B; de Bont, LGM; Boering, G. A proposed classification of temporomandibular disorders based on synovial joint pathology. J Craniomandib Pract (1989), 7:107–118.
3. Stegenga, B; de Bont, LGM; Boering, G. Osteoarthrosis as the cause of craniomandibular pain and dysfunction: A unifying concept. J Oral Maxillofac Surg (1989), 47:249–256.
4. de Bont, LGM; Boering, G; Liem, RSB; Havinga, P. Osteoarthritis of the temporomandibular joint: A light microscopic and scanning electron microscopic study of the articular cartilage of the mandibular condyle. J Oral Maxillofac Surg (1985), 43:481–488.
5. de Bont, LGM; Liem, RSB; Boering, G; et al. Osteoarthritis and internal derangement of the temporomandibular joint. A light microscopic study. J Oral Maxillofac Surg (1986), 44:634–643.
6. Johnson, LL. Normal arthroscopic findings of the patella. In: Arthroscopic Surgery. Principles and Practice. Vol II. St. Louis: CV Mosby Co. (1986), 816–823.

Two

Intracapsular Fibrosis Related to Pain and Dysfunction

RONALD M. KAMINISHI, D.D.S.

One of the major factors associated with temporomandibular joint (TMJ) dysfunction is the articular disk. Once considered the primary cause, the interarticular disk may only be part of the problem. The intracapsular etiology of TMJ dysfunction has and still is considered to be disk displacement with or without repositioning. The disk was considered a physical obstacle obstructing normal condylar translation when mandibular dysfunction occurred.

The etiology of TMJ pain continues to be controversial. One of the few common theories is that the cause of TMJ pain can be multifactorial.

In the 1980s new technology and techniques gave us more insight into TMJ pain and dysfunction. The purpose of this chapter is to discuss some of those discoveries.

Magnetic resonance imaging (MRI) has given us our first visual representation of the TMJ interarticular disk. Previous techniques showed a negative space from which we deduced data, or "computer-enhanced" images on a computer monitor, but did not provide a true representation of the disk. For the first time we can accurately image the position, shape, size, and consistency of the interarticular disk.

With MRI we have discovered that 30–40% of a "normal TMJ" population may have anterior disk displacement with or without reduction.[1]

With MRI we have learned that anterior disk displacement may not be present in TMJ dysfunctions such as closed-lock.[2] The disk that is anteriorly displaced and acting as a physical barrier may be only one reason translation is limited. We now know there

are other major factors in closed-lock dysfunction of the mandible—other factors limiting translation.

In an MRI survey taken on patients with TMJ dysfunction, it was demonstrated that the disk can be located in a number of different positions.[3] The disk position in such cases can range from a "normal" condyle-fossa relationship (Fig. 2–1) to total displacement beyond the articular eminence. In this group of patients there are MRIs in which the disk appears to be totally absent.

If the physical obstruction of the disk is not the only factor in TMJ dysfunction, what else is happening? What causes the disk to be anteriorly displaced? What causes closed-lock TMJ dysfunction if the disk is in the "normal" position when the mouth is closed? The answers begin to appear in the MRI with the mandible in the open position. The fact that the disk frequently remains in a fixed position becomes evident. This may occur in degrees. However, one can usually demonstrate that in both the closed and the open mouth positions, part or all of the disk remains fixed to a portion of the superior joint structures. Most commonly, this takes place in an area of the eminence, but it may occur in the fossa as well.

The question then arises as to why the disk is not moving. Why is it fixed in the same position? As other chapters in this book discuss, many new arthroscopic surgical techniques have evolved. All address intracapsular immobility. Some only minimally address disk position.

Use of the arthroscope has opened up new insights in TMJ pathology. With the ability to view the intra-

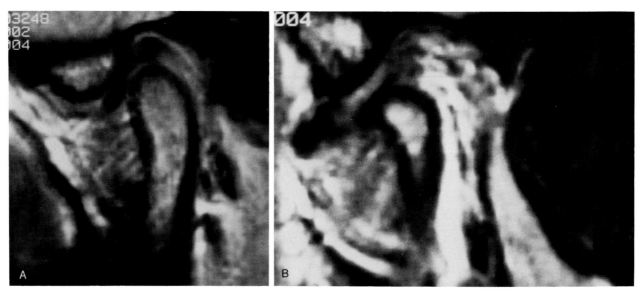

FIGURE 2–1. *A*—A magnetic resonance imaging (MRI) survey of closed-lock with the disk in the normal position (jaw closed). *B*—An MRI of closed-lock with the disk displaced beyond the eminence.

capsular environment in a more physiologic state, new information is available in TMJ pathophysiology. The arthroscope has provided a means of microsurgical evaluation with minimal destruction of joint structures.[15–18] A more precise picture of TMJ pathophysiology is evolving. The concept of recapturing, repositioning, replacing, substituting, or eliminating the articular disk may not be the ultimate goal of TMJ therapy. Evidence is growing that successful TMJ surgery may be performed without correcting disk position or function.[4,5]

In the overwhelming majority of patients with TMJ dysfunction, intracapsular fibrosis is encountered on arthroscopic examination of dysfunctional joints. Sometimes it ranges from thin filaments to heavy calcifying masses totally immobilizing the joint. This may occur within the superior or inferior joint spaces or may be associated with the capsule. In a small percentage of patients, arthroscopic release of fibrosis can result in proper repositioning of the disk and the reestablishment of translatory function.[4,6]

The following is a system to describe different categories to aid in better understanding this problem. Intracapsular, capsular, and extracapsular fibrosis appears to be a major factor in disk immobility.

SIMPLE FIBROUS BANDS (Fig. 2–2)

The simplest form of fibrosis is fibrous adhesions. These may range from lacy spider web–like threads to thick fibrous bands. Histologically, fibrous adhesions range from immature to very mature fibrous tissue. They usually connect the superior aspect of the joint compartment to the inferior aspect of the joint compartment. Superiorly, they are attached by means of the periosteum or articular cartilage to the fossa or eminences. Inferiorly, they may be attached to retrodiscal tissue, the disk, the pseudodisk, or the anterior bands.

The term "pseudodisk" is used to designate the

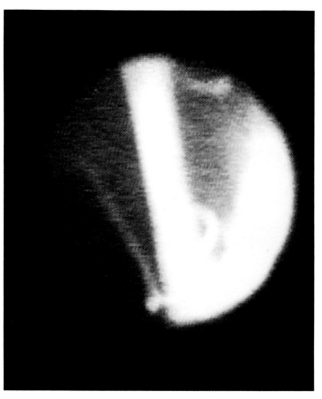

FIGURE 2–2. Simple fibrous bands.

adaptive retrodiscal tissue in the normal position of the disk when the true disk is displaced anteriorly, medially, or laterally. It is assumed for the rest of this chapter that all fibroses will be attached similarly to the upper and lower aspects of the superior joint space. As of the publication of this book, most arthroscopic study has been conducted in the upper compartment of the TMJ. Therefore, discussion is limited to the superior compartment.

How do these bands develop? The answer can only be theorized from current knowledge and observation. It is known that the normal joint is covered with articular cartilage in areas where articular forces are transmitted, i.e., the articular eminence and the head of the condyle. The rest of the joint is lined with synovial tissue. This is a very specialized tissue with specialized function, as is discussed in other chapters. We know that when there is abnormal joint function, such as micro- or macrotrauma, the synovium or sub-synovial tissue is easily injured. This very delicate tissue then rapidly undergoes the normal healing response. Of particular interest is the stage in which fibrin is formed by the underlying connective tissue. This, in turn, changes the surface of the synovium from a layer of synovial fluid overlying the synovial cells to a layer of fibrin.[7, 8] This changes a "super slippery" surface, designed for minimal to zero friction, to a "sticky" surface. This is most likely the etiology of the "suction cup" effect described as one of the findings in the etiology of TMJ closed-lock.[9] The surfaces adhere together and disk immobilization occurs. The fibrin then naturally becomes mature fibrous tissue.

Another theory implicates hematomas as the source of the fibrosis. There appears to be a high frequency of hematomas, subsynovial hyperemia, and ecchymosis found in the pathologic joint. When the hematomas are investigated closely, the normal sequence of transition to fibrin and fibrous tissue within these hematomas may be found. At times, immature fibrous bands can be seen separating as the arthroscope is manipulated in and around the mature hematomas present in the diseased joint.

FIBROSYNOVIAL BANDS (Fig. 2–3)

The fibrosynovial band has the same core as the simple fibrous band, except that the latter is covered by a layer of synovial tissue. This appears to be a progression of the simple fibrous band. Histologic studies show that the synovial cells at the base of these lesions proliferate and migrate across the fibrous tissue.[7] This would suggest a more mature lesion, possibly indicative of a more chronic problem.

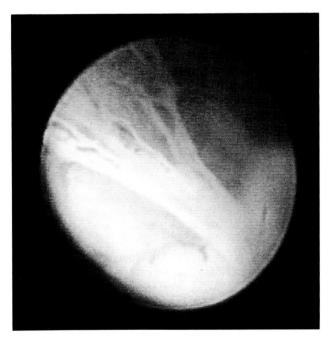

FIGURE 2–3. Fibrosynovial bands.

EARLY VERSUS LATE FIBROSIS

Occasionally, an area of distinct fibrosis between the eminence and the junction of the bilaminar zone and the disk or pseudodisk is encountered. If the area is in the early stage of transition from fibrin to mature fibrous tissue, the tissue may be very friable or soft. Positioning the scope for close inspection causes the tissues to spontaneously separate. Small areas of microhemorrhage can be seen. Sometimes the entire area of fibrosis can be resected by the arthroscopic examination alone. However, the resection may be very difficult if the tissues have matured.

CAPSULAR FIBROSIS (Fig. 2–4)

The normal capsule is seen arthroscopically as a homogeneous series of vertical or oblique fibers. An inferior vestibule is found on both the medial and the lateral capsules. In a pathologic capsule, distinct, thick bands of fibrous tissue, within or protruding from the capsule, may be observed. They are usually not parallel to the homogeneous fibers of the normal capsule, although this may also occur. This feature may be found in both the medial and the lateral capsules.

The fibrous bands may be very rigid when manipulated with a probe. In the presence of such fibrosis on the lateral capsule the lateral gutter along the inferior aspect is usually obliterated. This may be indicative of lateral capsular entrapment,[10] a condition in which the

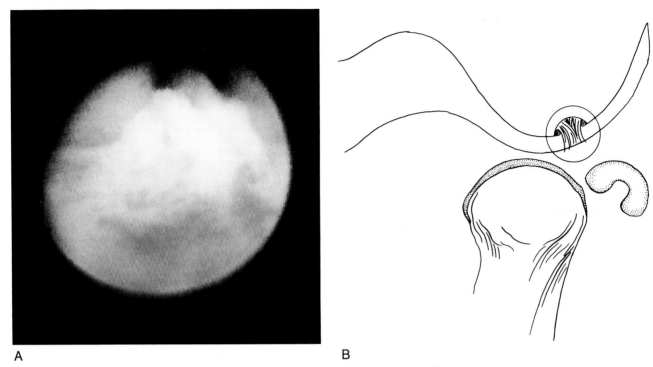

A   B

FIGURE 2–4. Capsular fibrosis. *A*—Arthroscopic photograph. *B*—Schematic drawing of *A*.

lateral capsule is retracted into the joint space as the disk rotates anteriorly and medially. This is accompanied by the sequence of tissue trauma, hemorrhage with or without surface fibrin exudation, combined with subsequent fibrous obliteration and immobilization. The intracapsular details of such lesions can only be seen arthroscopically. Thickened or partially fibrosed capsules are commonly encountered during arthrotomy. As they must be transected in the process of arthrotomy, their clinical significance has not been well understood. Arthroscopically transecting or stretching these restrictive bands contributes to the improvement of joint mobility and reduction of pain.[10]

DISK OSSEOUS BANDS
(Figs. 2–5 and 2–6)

This category describes a fibrous band attached to bone itself. In contrast, for almost all the other types of fibrosis described, the fibrotic tissue is attached to the cortical bone by means of the periosteum. The disk osseous band penetrates the cortical layer via an orifice in the cortical bone. Each band appears to have its own individual orifice. When the band is transected and the orifice explored, the origin of the fibrosis appears to be the medullary bone. This arthroscopic discovery may help to explain one of the etiologic factors of intracapsular pain. It is well known that there are few pain fibers within the TMJ, but it is also

well known that there are definite pain fibers in the bone.[11–13]

These bands have been observed primarily penetrating the articular eminence. They may vary in size.

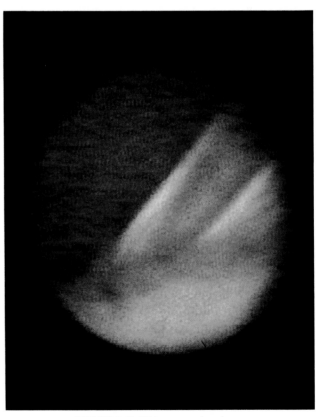

FIGURE 2–5. Disk osseous bands.

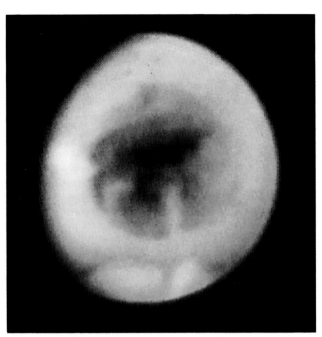

FIGURE 2–6. Osseous perforation in the eminence.

They may appear in isolation or in groups of as many as 10 or 12. Inferiorly, they have been observed attached to the adaptive bilaminar zone of the anterior displaced disk. Most consist of more delicate fibrous tissue and are easily resected.

PSEUDOWALLS

The term "pseudowall" is used to describe fibrous or fibrosynovial "walls" of tissue that partially or completely traverse the joint space from the medial to the lateral capsule. They are usually superiorly attached to the anterior slope, apex, or posterior slope of the eminence. The vast majority are found along the anterior slope of the eminence. Inferiorly, the wall is attached to the retrodiscal tissue, the disk, the pseudodisk, or the anterior band.

On the posterior aspect, pseudowalls appear to make a smooth transition to the surface where they are attached. The fibrous tissue gently curves between one structure and the next, whether the medial or the lateral capsule, the eminence, the retrodiscal tissue, the disk or the anterior band.

For yet unknown reasons, the body separates the superior joint space into one or more compartments by means of these pseudowalls. Pseudowalls are not normal anatomic findings but in fact are distinct pathologic entities; hence the description "false wall." During the learning curve of arthroscopic surgical orientation, one can and will be fooled by these false walls. They will completely partition a portion of the joint space, giving the illusion of a short joint.

Partial Fibrous and Fibrosynovial Pseudowalls (Fig. 2–7)

As their name implies, these walls only partially traverse the medial lateral dimension of the joint. They may start at either the medial or the lateral capsule. They connect the superior aspect to the inferior aspect of the joint spaces. The medial lateral dimension may vary. The maturity of the fibrous tissue within the wall may not be homogeneous. As with the fibrous bands, there may be a covering of synovial tissue with subsynovial vasculature covering the fibrous tissue.

Intermittent Fibrous and Fibrosynovial Pseudowalls

This form of pseudowall is composed of columns of fibrous bands that are usually wider than the simple fibrous bands. These intermittent columns alternate with open spaces. Superiorly and inferiorly, these columns are attached as mentioned earlier. They may be connected by sheets of synovial tissue. When viewed arthroscopically from a distance, alternating white and dark bands can be seen. The white bands are the fibrous tissue columns. The dark bands are the opening that continues into the anterior aspect of the joint. It must be remembered that without the scope light the joint appears dark. Only under close arthroscopic examination can a thin sheet of synovium sometimes be seen connecting the columns. If the inspection is done too vigorously, the synovium is easily obliterated.

Total Fibrous and Fibrosynovial Pseudowalls: Single and Multiple (Fig. 2–8)

As their names imply, these walls totally separate the superior joint space into different compartments. Most commonly, a simple wall separating the anterior recess from the rest of the joint is found. This wall is usually attached to the anterior slope near the apex of the eminence. Inferiorly, it may be attached to anteriorly displaced retrodiscal tissue, the disk, or the anterior band. The fibrous wall is composed of disorganized fibrous tissue. The posterior surface of the wall usually appears smooth. The surface appears as a homogeneous fibrous matrix sometimes formed apparently by parallel fibrous bands. However, on close inspection the fibrous tissue is haphazard in organization and thickness. There may be holes in the wall that appear as black spots. These holes are portals through which the dark anterior joint space can be seen.

The anterior surface of these walls varies from tissue totally covered by coagulated blood and hematoma to

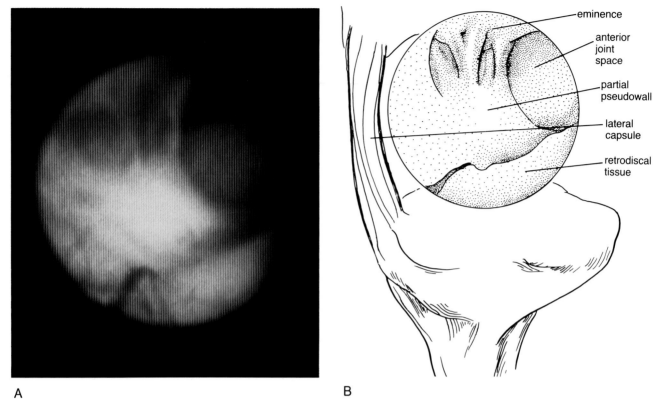

A
B

FIGURE 2–7. A partial fibrosynovial pseudowall. *A*—Arthroscopic photograph. *B*—Schematic drawing of *A*.

a very rough, chaotic-appearing aggregation of fibrous bands (Fig. 2–9). With the exception of a vertical partition, there usually does not appear to be any organized structure to this side of the wall. When the walls are transected, there is generally a significant amount of hemorrhage, demonstrating that vascular elements are present within this structure. There is also early evidence that peripheral neurologic struc-

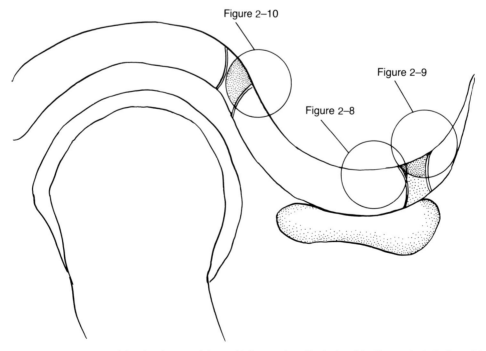

A schematic representation of the distribution of the multiple pseudowalls depicted in Figures 2–8, 2–9, and 2–10.

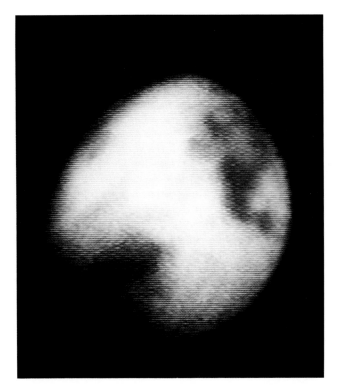

FIGURE 2–8. Posterior surface of a total fibrosynovial pseudowall.

tures are present within these pseudowalls.[14] This finding deserves further investigation.

The majority of these walls are covered on their posterior surfaces by a layer of synovium of varying thickness. The subsynovial vascularity and hyperemia vary greatly. The synovium on these walls usually presents various degrees of inflammation. The synovium appears to easily bridge voids or defects in the fibrous tissue. Thus, fibrosynovial pseudowalls usually present a homogeneous and uniform surface texture.

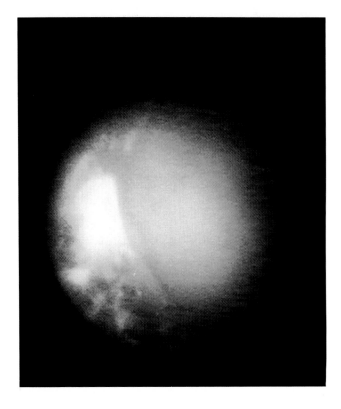

FIGURE 2–9. Anterior surface of a total fibrosynovial pseudowall, posterior slope of eminence.

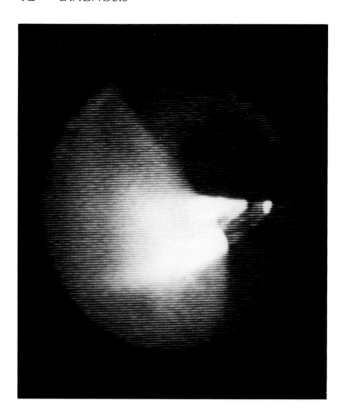

FIGURE 2–10. Anterior surface of a second pseudowall (same joint as in Fig. 2–8). Note the needle perforating through from the posterior recess.

Again, on close inspection the darker areas underlying the synovial layer reveal the inconsistencies of the fibrous tissue wall.

There have not been any observations or reports of a synovium covering the anterior aspect of any pseudowall.

More than one pseudowall can occur in the superior joint space. The posterior wall is found on the posterior

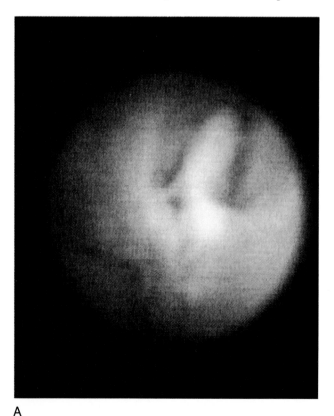

A

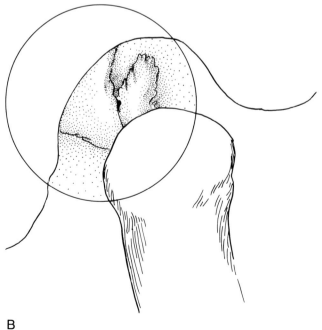

B

FIGURE 2–11. Interosseous fibrosis. A—Arthroscopic photograph. B—Schematic drawing of A.

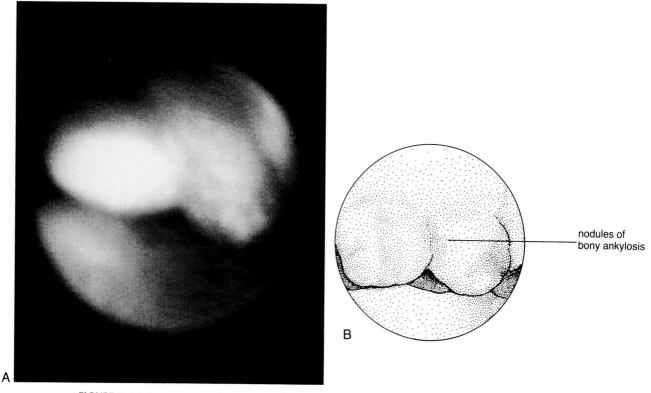

FIGURE 2–12. Posterior wall of bony ankylosis. *A*—Arthroscopic photograph. *B*—Schematic drawing of *A*.

slope of the eminence and is attached inferiorly to the retrodiscal tissue. The anterior wall is located along the anterior slope of the eminence and is usually attached inferiorly to the adapting retrodiscal tissue of the anteriorly displaced disk. Both anterior and posterior total pseudowalls traverse the joint from the medial to the lateral capsule. The body may separate the superior joint space into 3 distinct joint compartments (Fig. 2–10).

INTEROSSEOUS FIBROSIS (Fig. 2–11)

Chronic, severe TMJ disease may result in a large perforation or the obliteration of the interarticular disk. Perforations of this nature may expose the articulating surface of the condyle to the superior joint space.

Interosseous fibrosis may occur between the osseous elements of the fossa or the eminence and the condyle. This form of fibrosis usually consists of thick, very mature fibrous elements. They are attached to the bone of the eminence or the fossa and the condyle. Synovial coverings have not been observed in these types of lesions. Visualization of such pathosis under function shows how restrictive they are to the translation of the condyle.

FIBROOSSEOUS OR OSSEOUS ADHESIONS (Fig. 2–12)

These findings are more realistically referred to as fibroosseous ankylosis or bony ankylosis. When clearly diagnosed prior to treatment, they contraindicate arthroscopic procedures. Occasionally, in closed-lock dysfunction of the TMJ, bony ankylosis is indistinguishable from intracapsular fibrosis.

In the arthroscopic photograph in Figure 2–12, it appears as though fibrosynovial total pseudowall is present. However, when attempts were made in this case to transect the pseudowall, osseous elements were discovered. As the arthroscopic picture of the total fibrosynovial pseudowall is virtually identical to that found in bony ankylosis, it is speculated that there may be a strong correlation between these two types of lesions.

SUMMARY

Arthroscopy and MRI have shown that intracapsular fibrosis may be considered a major factor in TMJ pain and dysfunction. In the elective surgical ablation and débridement of such pathosis by means of arthroscopic surgery, reestablishment of translatory function in the superior disk space is accomplished. This is accompanied by significantly increased opening and improved function. Studies show this is accomplished with or without normalizing disk position, disk function, or both, in the majority of cases.

It has also been shown that ablation and débridement of intracapsular fibrosis may significantly reduce pain.[2, 10] Periosteal pain fibers and osseous pain fibers play a significant role in pain associated with other parts of the body. It has been submitted that they play a significant role in pain of the TMJ. The range from simple fibrous adhesions to complete osseous ankylosis has also been described. The challenge that has been presented is to use this added information in the continuing search for the true pathophysiology of TMJ disease.

REFERENCES

1. Kircos, LT; et al. Magnetic resonance imaging of the TMJ disc on asymptomatic volunteers. J Oral Maxillofac Surg (1987), 45:852–854.
2. Davis, CL; Kaminishi, RM; Burnett, K. TMJ Arthroscopy and MR Imaging. California Dental Association Journal (1988), 16:52–56.
3. Kaminishi, RM; Davis, CL. Classification of disc position in closed lock. In preparation for publication.
4. Moses, J; et al. The effect of arthroscopic surgery lysis and lavage of the superior joint space on TMJ disc position and mobility. J Oral Maxillofac Surg (1989), 47:674–678.
5. Perrott, DH; Alborzi, A; et al. A prospective evaluation of the effectiveness of temporomandibular joint arthroscopy. J Oral Maxillofac Surg (1990), 48:1029–1032.
6. Montgomery, MT; Van Sickels, J; et al. Arthroscopic TMJ surgery: Effects on signs, symptoms, and disc position. J Oral Maxillofac Surg (1989), 47:1263–1271.
7. Kao, R; Lee, C. Synovial lesions. Lecture presented at the Craniomandibular Institute, Squaw Valley, California, January 1989.
8. Soren, A. Histodiagnosis and Clinical Correlation of Rheumatoid and Other Synovitis. Philadelphia: JB Lippincott Co. (1978).
9. Sanders, B; Buoncristiani, R. Diagnostic and surgical arthroscopy of the TMJ: Clinical experience with 137 patients over 2 years. J Craniomandib Dis Fac Oral Pain (1987), 1:202–213.
10. Moses, J. Personal communication regarding lateral capsular entrapment. January, 1989.
11. Hohmann, EL; Elde, RP; Rysavy, JA; et al. Innervation of periosteum and bone by sympathetic vasoactive intestinal peptide-containing nerve fibers. Science (1986), 232:868–871.
12. Tanaka, S; Ito, T. Histochemical demonstration of adrenergic fibers in the fascia periosteum and retinaculum. Clin Orthopedics (1987), 126:276–281.
13. Sakada, S; Maeda, K. Characteristics of innervation and nerve ending in CAT mandibular periosteum. Bull Tokyo Dent Coll (1967), 8:77–84.
14. Kaminishi, RM. Early biopsy evidence. Case Study: Biopsy of Intraarticular Pseudowall. June 1988 to present.
15. Ohnishi, M. Arthroscopy of the temporomandibular joint. [in Japanese]. Kokubyo Gakkai Zasshi (1975), 42:207–213.
16. Dandy, DJ. Arthroscopy of the Knee. London, England: Gower Medical Publishing Ltd. (1984).
17. Johnson, L. Arthroscopic Surgery. St. Louis: CV Mosby Co. (1986).
18. Oral Maxillofac Surg Clin North Am: Disorders of the TMJ (1989), 1:1–151.

Three

Intraarticular Adhesions of the Temporomandibular Joint
Arthroscopic Views and Clinical Perspectives

KEN-ICHIRO MURAKAMI, D.D.S., PH.D.
NATSUKI SEGAMI, D.D.S., PH.D.

Intraarticular fibrous adhesion is one of the important pathologic signs of intracapsular temporomandibular joint (TMJ) diseases, but this factor has been rarely described with respect to its arthroscopic characteristics[1,2] and cadaveric histology.[3] The purposes of this chapter are (1) to describe the incidence and distribution of fibrous adhesions in patients with internal derangement and arthrosis, and (2) to describe the correlation between adhesions and the clinical subjective symptoms of patients with internal derangement of the TMJ with closed-lock.

ARTHROSCOPIC FINDINGS OF ADHESIONS IN CONSECUTIVE CASES

In order to explore adhesions in intracapsular TMJ diseases, 68 consecutive arthroscopically examined TMJs were evaluated in 56 patients (8 males and 48 females) ranging in age from 15 to 69 years, with an average age of 32.7 years. The clinical diagnoses were internal derangement with clicking in 6 joints, internal derangement with closed-lock in 30 joints, degenerative joint disease (DJD) in 9 joints, and closed-lock combined with DJD change in 23 joints (Table 3–1). With the patient under general or local anesthesia, upper joint compartment arthroscopy was performed and systematically observed using the single or multiportal approaches described previously.[4,5] The examination of adherent pathology was done by both direct arthroscopic inspection and a probing technique (palpation) using a hooked or straight probe (Fig. 3–1).

On the basis of pathologic arthroscopy, adhesions were classified as being one of 3 types: a band-like adhesion, a filmy adhesion, or a pseudowall adhesion. A band-like adhesion was identified as a fibrous band connecting the intersynovial structures, from the roof to the bottom structure (Fig. 3–2). This pathology was observed both in the anterior and posterior synovial pouch or recess, and usually in the medial capsular area (Fig. 3–3). The second type, the filmy adhesion, was defined as surface stickiness between the articular surfaces of the temporal component and the articular

TABLE 3–1. PREOPERATIVE DIAGNOSES AND NUMBER OF SUBJECTS

Internal derangements	
Click	6
Closed-lock	30
DJD*	9
Closed-lock with DJD	23
Total	68 TMJs† in 56 patients

*Degenerative joint disease.
†Temporomandibular joint.

15

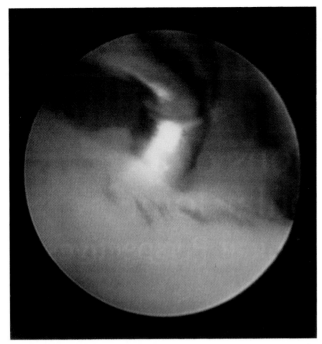

FIGURE 3–1. Diagnostic arthroscopy by means of the probing technique to detect the degree of restriction by the adhesion.

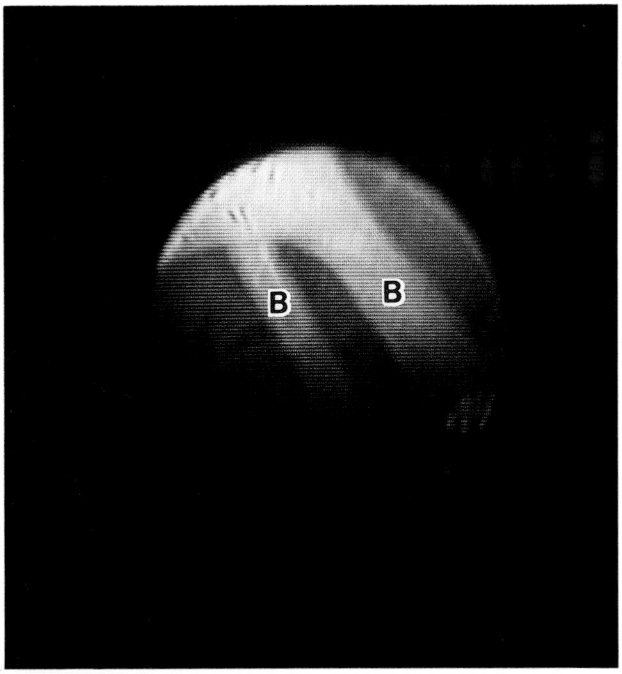

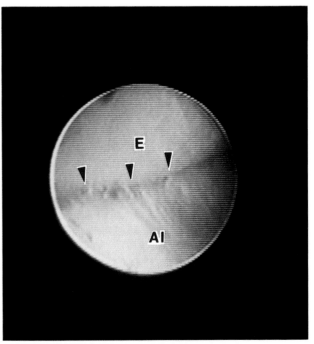

FIGURE 3–3. Band-like adhesion between the eminence and the posterior attachment located on the intermediate zone (B: adhesion).

disk or posterior disk attachment (Fig. 3–4). This adhesion was usually detected in the intermediate space between the articular eminence and the articular disk or posterior attachment. The third type, the pseudowall adhesion, was commonly observed in the anterolateral aspect of the upper joint cavity (Figs. 3–5 and 3–6). As this type of broad adhesion is frequently formed at

the anterior boundaries of the upper joint cavity, distinguishing the real capsule from this structure is not easy (Fig. 3–7). Under close examination, however, loss of the direction of fiber texture on the adhesion surface is revealed, as is the irregular distri-

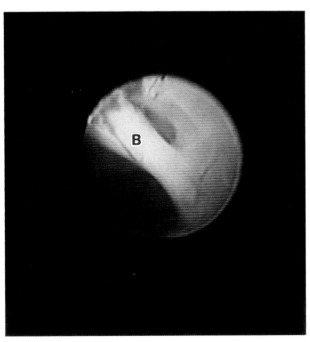

FIGURE 3–2. Band-like adhesion in the anterior recess (B: adhesion).

FIGURE 3–4. Filmy adhesion on the posterolateral aspect of the eminence (E: eminence; Al: lateral attachment of the disk; *arrows*: adhesion).

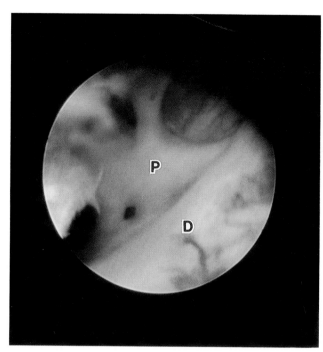

FIGURE 3–5. Pseudowall in the anterior recess of the right temporomandibular joint (D: anteriorly displaced disk; P: pseudowall).

bution of capillary networks, such as in scar tissue. For precise and appropriate observation and palpation of this pseudowall in the anterior recess, an optional arthroscopic approach, such as anterolateral puncture, endaural puncture, or both may be a useful addition to the conventional first puncture.

Based on the observation of 68 consecutive cases,

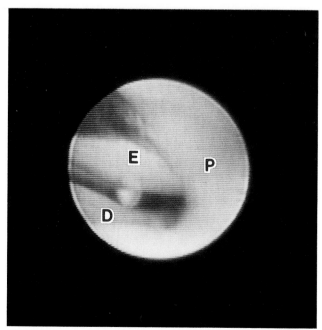

FIGURE 3–6. Pseudowall located close to the lateral capsule of the right temporomandibular joint (E: eminence; D: disk; P: pseudowall).

the overall incidence of intraarticular adhesion was 91.2% (62 of the 68 joints examined displayed some form of adherent pathology). Pseudowall adhesion was the predominant pathology (80.9%, or 55 of 68 joints), followed by filmy adhesion (41.2%, or 28 joints) and band-like adhesion (22.1%, or 15 joints). Some types of adhesion were found to overlap.

When the group with derangement with clicking was compared with the other groups, the other groups were found to have a greater incidence of adhesions. The groups with DJD and closed-lock combined with DJD change had cases presenting with some form of adhesion.

The distribution and detection of the three types of adhesion differed in each of the diagnostic subgroups. In the group with clicking, no pseudowall formation was found, and there was only a low incidence of band-like and filmy adhesions (2 of 6 joints in each case). In the closed-lock cases, the predominant type of adhesion was the pseudowall, which was observed in 28 of all 30 joints (93.3%), followed by filmy adhesion (in 7 of 30) and band-like adhesion (in 4 of 30). In the cases with DJD, however, the most frequently observed form was the filmy adhesion (in all of the 9 joints), followed by the pseudowall (in 7 of 9 joints), and the band-like adhesion (in 3 of 9 joints). The cases of closed-lock with DJD change had a high incidence of pseudowall adhesion (87.0%, or 20 of 23 joints), and a low incidence of band-like adhesion (26.1%, or 6 of 23 joints), and a moderate incidence of filmy adhesion (52.2%, or 12 of 23 joints). The incidence of filmy adhesion appeared to have a tendency to increase when it was associated with DJD change (Table 3–2).

The pathogenesis and etiology of intraarticular adhesion have not been elucidated. Kaminishi and Davis[1] hypothesized the formation of adhesions in the TMJ based on the orthopedic literature. One theory is that synovitis causes fibrin deposition, which decreases joint lubrication. The resultant suction cup effect and immobilized joint causes the fibrin deposition to continue, with the formation of fibrous adhesions. Another theory is that hematomas in the synovial membrane attract

TABLE 3–2. INCIDENCE AND DISTRIBUTION OF EACH TYPE OF FIBROUS ADHESION

Internal Derangement	Band-like Adhesion	Pseudowall	Filmy Adhesion	Number of TMJs* with Adhesions
Click	2/6	0/6	2/6	2/6
Closed-lock	4/30	28/30	7/30	28/30
DJD†	6/23	20/23	12/23	23/23
DJD with closed-lock	3/9	7/9	9/9	9/9
Total	15/68	55/68	28/68	62/68

*Temporomandibular joint.
†Degenerative joint disease.

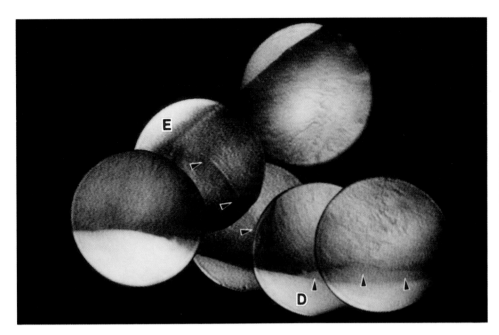

FIGURE 3–7. Pseudowall formation from medial to anterior capsule of the right temporomandibular joint (E: eminence; D: disk; arrows: adhesion).

fibroblasts and fibrocytes to the area. The healing process results in the formation of scar tissue on the existing fibrous capsular wall.

The pseudowall adhesion may be explained by the latter condition. Mechanical squeezing of the synovium in the anterior recess due to anterior disk displacement results in the folding and fusion of the synovial membrane (Fig. 3–8) combined with hematoma formation or with microbleeding in cases of inflammation. The plicate synovium incorporates with the capsular wall to form scar tissue. Pseudowall adherence was only observed in the anterior synovial recess and the anterolateral aspect of the upper joint cavity. In addition, the surface characteristics of this adhesion are similar to those of a scar. Usually, a histopathologic specimen shows degenerative fibrous connective tissue combined

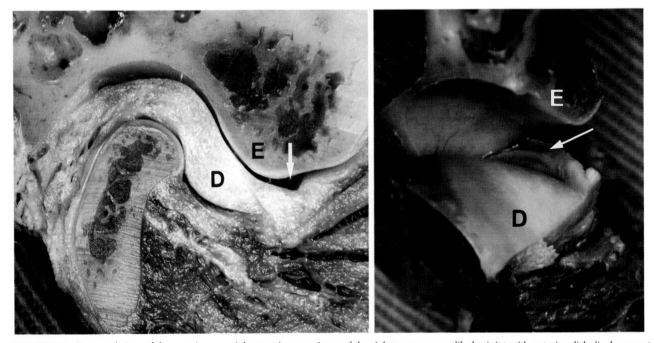

FIGURE 3–8. Dissected view of the anterior synovial recess in a specimen of the right temporomandibular joint with anterior disk displacement without reduction. *Left*: sagittal section; *right*: anterior synovial recess viewed from posterior to anteromedial aspect. The synovial membrane is compressed and folded presumably due to disk displacement *(arrows)* (D: articular disk; E: articular eminence).

TABLE 3–3. PATIENT BACKGROUND

28 patients:	Age: 31.9 ± 17.5 years old
Male 2	Opening degree: 27.9 ± 5.2 mm
Female 26	Locking duration: 9.4 ± 13.1 months

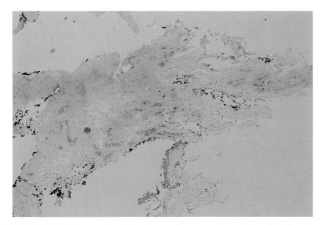

FIGURE 3–9. Histopathologic view of removed pseudowall adhesion.

with mild inflammatory cell infiltrate and fine vascular proliferation (Fig. 3–9).

The band-like adhesion may result in part from this pathophysiology. However, the filmy adhesion cannot be explained by the hematoma–scar formation theory, and it is insufficiently explained by the fibrin deposition theory described earlier. As long as the synovial cells are functioning, fibrin and other products are phagocytosed. The decrease in viscosity and the reduced joint lubrication that result in the secondary suction cup effect may be closely related to the pathogenesis of chondromalacia. Quinn[6, 7] has described the sequential pathogenesis of degenerative changes of articular cartilage, the destruction of the cartilaginous matrix, presumably due to overloading or joint malalignment and involving disk derangement, and the release of cathepsin and other collagenases. Cathepsin and other collagenases increase synovial vascular permeability, reduce synovial fluid viscosity (owing to synovial fluid's high plasma protein content) and accelerate the production of chemical pain mediators via the synovium. Fibrillation and softening of the cartilage increase joint friction. Thus, in this stage, fibrin deposition may play a role in articular immobilization, which subsequently leads to fibrous maturation. Our observations have shown that filmy adhesion is much more evident in cases with DJD change. This suggests that the hypothesis that the pathophysiology of filmy adhesion is based on the previous explanation is reasonable.

CORRELATION BETWEEN INTRAARTICULAR ADHESIONS AND CLINICAL SYMPTOMS

In order to study the correlation between the adhesions and clinical symptoms, such as the limited range of mandibular motion as well as the subjective feeling of a locking jaw, both the arthroscopic findings of

adhesion and questionnaires on subjective jaw function were quantitatively scored and evaluated.

Twenty-eight of the female and two of the male patients participated in this study. Using preoperative diagnostic imaging (magnetic resonance imaging or arthrography) all patients were diagnosed as having TMJ internal derangement with closed-lock (25 unilateral cases, 3 bilateral cases). Patient age ranged from 13 to 77 years and averaged 31.9 years. The degree of opening ranged from 13 mm to 36 mm and averaged 27.9 mm. The duration of the symptoms of locking ranged from 1 to 36 months and averaged 9.4 months (Table 3–3).

In order to grade intraarticular adhesion, the arthroscopic findings of adhesions were evaluated by means of an adhesion index quantifying both intensity (Table 3–4) and distribution. To examine the intensity, probing (palpation) was carried out in addition to arthroscopic inspection. Two surgeons discussed the grade of adhesion preoperatively and recorded it on the chart immediately after the operation (Fig. 3–10).

Jaw function was rated using a 57-item questionnaire. Each item required the patients to rate function on a scale from 0 to 4 points (Table 3–5). The degree of interincisal opening (in millimeters) was used to objectively represent the range of jaw motion.

Spearman's rank correlation coefficients of the adhesion indices and jaw function scores as well as of the degree of opening were tested. The hypothesis of no statistical difference was rejected if the probability level was less than or equal to .05.

In question one ("Do your joints make noise so that it bothers you or others?"), both the intensity and the distribution of adhesions correlated negatively. The distribution of adhesions and the degree of opening also correlated negatively but to a lesser degree. All

TABLE 3–4. SCALE OF INTENSITY OF ADHESION

Grade	Findings
0	No adhesion, no fibrous changes
1	Filmy adhesion (mild)
2	(moderate to severe)
3	Fibrosynovial band (mild to moderate)
4	(severe)
5	Fibrous band (mild to moderate)
6	(severe)
7	Pseudocapsular wall (mild to moderate)
8	(severe)
9	Capsular fibrosis (mild to moderate)
10	(severe)

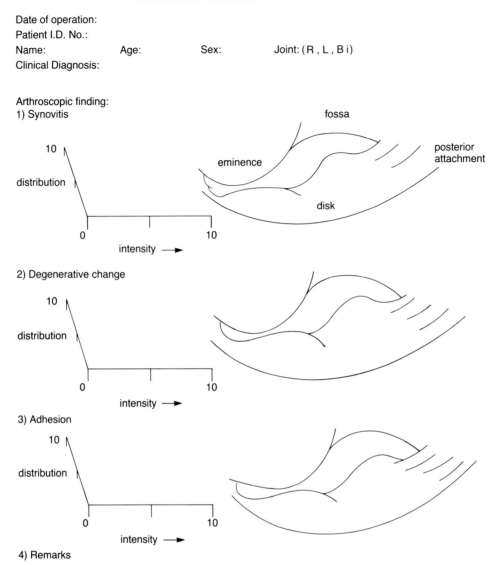

FIGURE 3–10. Arthroscopic operative record of pathologic findings.

other subjective symptoms, such as "difficult to open mouth wide," did not correlate with the adhesion indices or were statistically insignificant (Table 3–6).

As indicated by the optional data, the duration of closed-lock correlated significantly with both the intensity and the distribution of adhesions (0.561 and 0.638). The distribution of adhesions and patient age also correlated (0.428).

The data obtained revealed that the correlation between intraarticular adhesion and the signs and symptoms of joint hypomobility was in general unexpectedly low. A weak but significant negative correlation between adherent distribution and degree of opening was found. More so than its intensity, the distribution of an adhesion seems to play a role in jaw hypomobility in closed-lock. A negative relationship

TABLE 3–5. JAW FUNCTION QUESTIONNAIRE

Jaw Function Questions	No	Maybe a Little	Quite a Lot	Almost All the Time	All the Time Without Stopping
1. Do your jaw joints make noise so that it bothers you or others?					
2. Do you find it difficult to open your mouth wide?					
3. Does your jaw ever get stuck (lock) as you open it?					
4. Does your jaw ever lock open so you cannot close it?					
5. Is your bite uncomfortable?					

TABLE 3–6. CORRELATION COEFFICIENTS BETWEEN INTRAARTICULAR ADHESIONS AND JAW FUNCTION

Jaw Function	Adhesion Intensity	Distribution
Jaw joints make noise	−0.458*	−0.484*
Jaw is difficult to open	−0.183	−0.276
Jaw gets stuck (locks)	0.132	−0.075
Jaw locks open	0.233	0.212
Biting is uncomfortable	0.164	0.332
Total jaw function	−0.105	−0.147
Degree of opening	−0.334	−0.393*

*$p < .05$

between the degree of joint murmur and adhesion was found, but the average score for this question was low. These results suggest that the adhesion may not be a significant barometer of joint hypomobility. Joint compartment volume or vertical tightness of joint play should be evaluated and may be managed and maintained by the lateral ligament. Clinical experience supports the usefulness of lateral release in the upper joint compartment (together with surgical lysis of adhesions) to unlock and mobilize the jaw in patients with closed-lock.[8] This indicates that the adhesion should be swept, but the adhesion may be associated with concomitant pathology in TMJ closed-lock. The essential pathogenesis of hypomobility is not addressed here. Apparently, disk position plays a small role in the explanation of this matter as has been verified by diagnostic imaging studies conducted after both conventional and arthroscopic surgery.[9,10]

The correlation of both the duration of locking and patient age with adhesion was addressed in this study. The findings were in agreement with the observations of adhesions in the cases described at the beginning of this chapter.

Regarding the relationship between pain and adhesions, Spearmann's rank correlation coefficient for the values of these factors was tested and found to indicate a weak correlation. Pain was found to have a greater relationship to the synovitis index than it did to the adhesion index. The details of this phenomenon are not addressed here.

SUMMARY

Various intraarticular adhesions are frequently detected in the superior joint compartment in patients with internal derangement and arthrosis of the TMJ. Adhesion type may be described as band-like, filmy, or pseudowall, and adhesion incidence has a tendency to increase with the duration of symptoms and patient age. The relationship between clinical signs and symptoms is reflected more in the degree of distribution of adhesions than in each intensity level. Correlations between subjective symptoms are, however, generally low. The adhesions might be considered as a concomitant disease in cases of intracapsular TMJ pathology.

REFERENCES

1. Kaminishi, RM; Davis, CL. Temporomandibular joint arthroscopic observations of superior space adhesions. Oral Maxillofac Surg Clin N Am (1989), 1:103–109.
2. Segami, N; Murakami, K; Fujimura, K; et al. Arthroscopic findings of internal derangement with closed lock of the temporomandibular joint [in Japanese]. Kokubyo Gakkai Zasshi (1989), 38:857–869.
3. Kurita, K; Bronstein, SL; Westesson, PL; et al. Arthroscopic diagnosis of perforation and adhesions of the temporomandibular joint: Correlation with postmortem morphology. Oral Surg Oral Med Oral Pathol (1989), 68:130–134.
4. Murakami, K; Ono, T. Temporomandibular joint arthroscopy by inferolateral approach. Int J Oral Maxillofac Surg (1986), 15:410–417.
5. McCain, JP; de la Rua, H. Principles and practice of operative arthroscopy of the human temporomandibular joint. Oral Maxillofac Surg Clin N Am (1989), 1:135–151.
6. Quinn, JH. Pathogenesis of temporomandibular joint chondromalacia and arthralgia. Oral Maxillofac Surg Clin N Am (1989), 1:47–57.
7. Quinn, JH. Identification of prostaglandin E_2 and leukotriene B_4 in the synovial fluid of painful, dysfunctional temporomandibular joints. J Oral Maxillofac Surg (1990), 48:968–971.
8. Moses, JJ. Lateral impingement syndrome and eudaural surgical technique. Oral Maxillofac Surg Clin N Am (1989), 1:165–183.
9. Moses, JJ; Sartoris, D; Glass, R; et al. The effect of arthroscopic surgical lysis and lavage of the superior joint space on TMJ disc position and mobility. J Oral Maxillofac Surg (1989), 47:674–678.
10. Montgomery, M; Van Sickels, JE; Harms, SE; Thrash, WJ. Signs and symptoms following TMJ meniscal repositioning surgery. J Dent Res (1989), 68:310.

Four

Arthroscopic Evaluation of Patients with Temporary Silastic Implants

JEROLD S. GOLDBERG, D.D.S.
JOHN F. DiSTEFANO, D.D.S.

The use of arthroscopy in the temporomandibular joint (TMJ) has aided the diagnosis and management of TMJ problems. It has also led to an increase in our knowledge and understanding of joint function and disease. This advanced technology, which allows for the examination of internal structures through small access portals, may have potential applications in patient care other than those usually described.

Arthroscopy has now been used in a somewhat unconventional manner to evaluate the TMJ following the placement of temporary Silastic implants at the time of implant removal, providing valuable information about how the TMJ is structurally responding to treatment. The surgical technique being investigated was first described by Dr. Clyde Wilkes in the late 1970s.[1] This technique is usually indicated in cases of late-stage disease in which the interarticular disk has been removed. Following disk removal, a piece of Silastic is fashioned to the approximate size and shape of a disk with a "tail" emanating from its lateral aspect. The disk portion is sutured with resorbable sutures to the lateral pterygoid muscle anteriorly and to the remnants of the retrodiscal pad posteriorly (Fig. 4–1). The "tail" portion is sutured just below the skin in front of the tragus (Fig. 4–2). At a later time, 1 to 4 months postoperatively, the "tail" is uncovered through a small opening in the original incision and the entire implant is removed. Preformed implants of higher density Silastic are now commercially available.

It has been hypothesized that a fibrous tissue capsule will form around this temporary implant and that this will aid in the healing of the articular surfaces of the condyle and glenoid fossa. It is also suggested that this temporary implant may prevent the vertical formation of adhesions between these osseous structures. Many surgeons have observed smooth, white, fibrous tissue covering the joint surfaces when long-term Silastic implants have been removed for a variety of reasons. A review of the literature finds no description of the lining surfaces of the joint at the time of removal of temporary Silastic implants.

Therefore, 11 TMJs in 9 patients were evaluated arthroscopically at the time of Silastic implant removal. All patients had a preoperative diagnosis of internal derangement. The diagnosis was based on clinical examination and confirmed with an imaging study. All patients had undergone unsuccessful nonsurgical treatment. Diagnostic blocks relieved pain. Temporary implants were placed when the disk was removed because structural alterations made repair of the disk impossible.

Implants were removed 1 to 4 months after placement. Indications for the exact time of implant removal were somewhat arbitrary. If patients developed joint noise other than the characteristic squeaky noise usual in this procedure, the implants tended to be removed early. Two patients were lost to follow-up; their implants were removed later than desired, at 8 and 16 months, respectively.

At the time of implant removal, a 1.9-mm arthro-

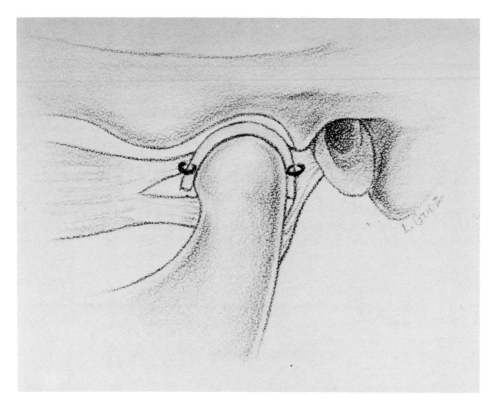

FIGURE 4–1. Silastic implant sutured to the lateral pterygoid muscle and the posterior attachments.

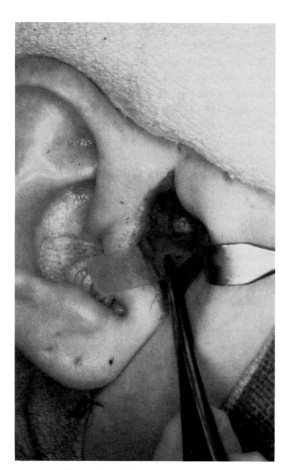

FIGURE 4–2. The "tail" of the implant prior to suture into the subcutaneous tissues.

scope was placed into the "fistula" created by the implant, and the joint space was examined (Fig. 4–3). A pursestring suture was placed around the arthroscope and near the wound edge in order to allow for joint distention with irrigation (Fig. 4–4).

It was possible to adequately examine the "fistula" leading into the joint and the space within the joint created by the implant. In all cases, there was soft tissue covering both the mandibular condyle and the glenoid fossa. The "fistula" leading to the joint area was always smooth, white, and glistening and had few or no blood vessels (Fig. 4–5). In the 7 patients who had implants removed at 4 months or earlier, the condyle and temporal bones were covered with smooth, glistening, pink tissue with few vessels. The tissue conformed to the contours of the Silastic and underlying bony structures (Fig. 4–6). In some joints there were small areas of tissue proliferation that may represent foreign body reactions or synovitis. In the 2 joints with an extended time interval (over 4 months) before implant removal, the appearance of the soft tissue was very different. The tissue appeared erythematous and intruded into the created joint space. The tissue did not follow the contours of the Silastic or the underlying bone.

DISCUSSION

This investigation demonstrates that a fibrous capsule forms around a Silastic implant placed in a TMJ

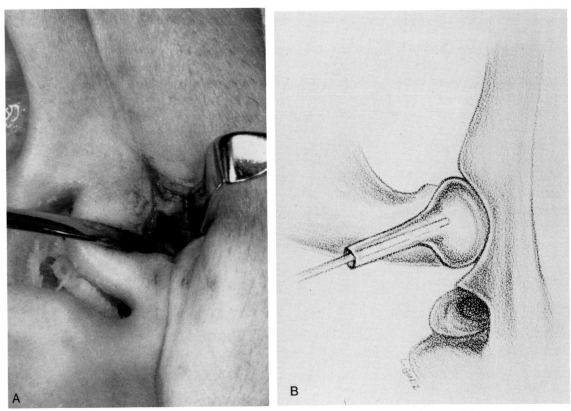

FIGURE 4–3. *A*—Fistula created by the "tail" of the implant at the time of removal. *B*—Schematic diagram of the entire fistula created by the implant as it is negotiated by an arthroscope.

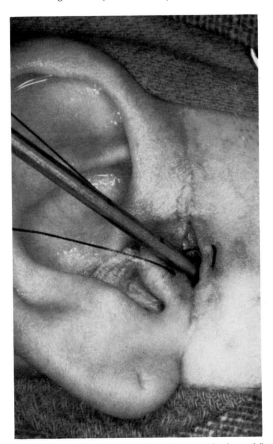

FIGURE 4–4. Purse-string suture used to decrease the loss of fluid for distension and the loss of light.

in the manner described by Wilkes. The quality of the covering tissue observed at the time of implant removal was generally encouraging. It must be noted, however, that our patients are restricted to a diet requiring no chewing for 3 months after the procedure; they only start to eat a soft diet at the time of implant removal. It is unknown how these tissues will react with the implant out of place and when the patient's diet has advanced to normal. The strict adherence to a diet requiring no chewing may also explain why the results in our patients seem somewhat more favorable than those described in other papers.[2,3]

It was noted that most implants showed some signs of wear. It must, therefore, be assumed that some Silastic particles may be in these joints. However, the significance of a small amount of Silastic in a joint is not well understood. Clearly, an extensive foreign body reaction is not desirable. On the other hand, Silastic implants have remained in place for many years in many joints without problems. Therefore, it seems reasonable that a small amount of Silastic does not create a clinically significant foreign body reaction.

It would be helpful if we could examine these joints arthroscopically and determine the best time for implant removal. Leaving implants in for over 4 months does not, in our experience, seem to be productive. With more experience, it may be that the ideal time for implant removal may be determined based on

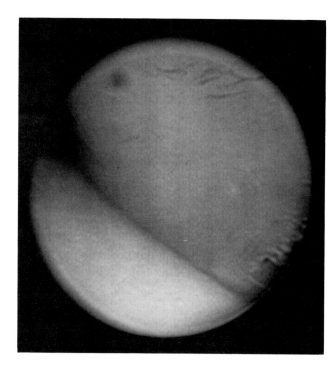

FIGURE 4–5. Arthroscopic picture of the "fistula" leading to the joint area.

averages or on arthroscopic observation. A correlation among the time of implant removal (in the 1- to 4-month group), the quality of tissue, and how patients are progressing was not accomplished.

It is also possible that arthroscopic intervention at the time of implant removal may influence results. Smoothing out small areas of irregularity may be helpful. It would be interesting to know if there is a relationship between the findings of an arthroscopic examination and the clinical course of the patient after implant removal.

In both cases in which implants were left in for an extended period of time, the patients required repeat surgery. At the time of the repeat surgery, a biopsy showed the anticipated foreign body reaction to what is, in all likelihood, Silastic fragments.

It is not the purpose of this chapter to advocate temporary Silastic implants as a preferred treatment for internal derangement, but rather to describe a new application of arthroscopic technique. These techniques may also be useful as an adjunct to other types of joint surgery.

Perhaps the arthroscopic examination of failed or failing open surgical procedures may allow for in-

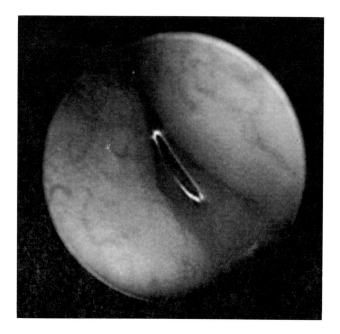

FIGURE 4–6. Arthroscopic picture demonstrating smooth tissues that conform to the contour of the osseous structures and the implant.

creased knowledge about causes of failure. It may be possible to intervene and salvage failing procedures using arthroscopic manipulations.

Other uses of the technique may include the examination of infected sites through an existing fistula. The examination of an infected bone plate may aid in decisions about its removal. The examination of bone in the case of osteomyelitis may be helpful in the timing of sequestrectomy.

We hope the investigation presented and the possible applications of arthroscopy suggested will encourage practitioners to consider other uses of this technology that may benefit patients.

REFERENCES

1. Wilkes, C. Personal communication, May 1980.
2. Eriksson, L; Westesson, PL. Deterioration of temporary silicone implant in the temporomandibular joint: A clinical and arthroscopic follow-up study. Oral Surg Oral Med Oral Pathol (1986), 62:2–6.
3. Dolwick, M; Aufdemarte, T. Silicone induced foreign body reaction and lymph-adenopathy after temporomandibular joint arthroplasty. Oral Surg Oral Med Oral Pathol (1985), 59:449–452.

PART 2

Treatment

Five

A 5-Year Experience with Arthroscopic Lysis and Lavage for the Treatment of Painful Temporomandibular Joint Hypomobility

BRUCE SANDERS, D.D.S.
RALPH BUONCRISTIANI, D.D.S.

Arthroscopic lysis and lavage is one type of operative arthroscopy of the temporomandibular joint (TMJ). It seems safe to conclude when conversing with surgeons and reviewing the many publications released and the scientific presentations made addressing arthroscopy that lysis and lavage is the most widely utilized form of TMJ operative arthroscopic surgery.[1-11]

Several lectures and abstracts presented at the 1988 and 1989 International TMJ Arthroscopic Symposia[12-14] showed excellent success rates for this simple procedure.[15,16] Available publications presenting large series of patients and good follow-up also show similarly good results. Two presentations made at the Symposia compared arthroscopy and open TMJ surgery (arthrotomy). The researchers had obtained at least equal results when they compared arthroscopy with arthrotomic disk repair procedures.[17,18]

It should be noted that arthroscopic lysis and lavage does not typically result in reduction of the anteriorly displaced disk. However, it does increase disk mobility and dramatically improve clinical symptoms.[6-8,11,14,16]

As of 1990, our experience with arthroscopic lysis and lavage has spanned 5 years. It was our intention not to vary our technique significantly so that we would be able to obtain a long-term exposure to this operative procedure.

When we observed the magnificent technical accomplishments of our surgical colleagues in the application of sophisticated cautery and suturing procedures and in the use of lasers, we were very much impressed. We are in awe of the tremendous surgical dexterity and the ingenuity in our colleagues' use of tiny manual cutting tools and motorized instruments. This is truly great work! However, no matter how far we may progress with exciting, new procedures and innovative technology in advanced operative arthroscopy, the results of each new technique will probably be compared with those obtained with lysis and lavage. This is why it is important to understand the strengths, the weaknesses, and the limitations of arthroscopic lysis and lavage. In this chapter we present a subjective clinical analysis evaluating this procedure. There are obvious flaws associated with this type of study, but hopefully our findings will provide some valuable information.

31

TABLE 5–1. RELATIONSHIP BETWEEN PATIENT AGE AND SEX AND THE AVERAGE DURATION OF SYMPTOMS*

Range in Age (years)	Male Patients	Female Patients	Average Duration of Symptoms	
			Years	Months
10–19	2	27	2	7
20–29	5	65	2	4
30–39	6	69	4	0
40–49	2	26	3	8
50–59	0	10	4	2
≥60	0	1	1	0
Totals	15	198	3	2

*Age and sex distribution as it relates to the average duration of symptoms in 213 patients undergoing arthroscopic surgery of the temporomandibular joint.

TABLE 5–2. RELATIONSHIP BETWEEN PATIENT AGE AND PREOPERATIVE DIAGNOSIS*

Range in Age (years)	Internal Derangements	Degenerative Joint Disease
10–19	27	2
20–29	52	17
30–39	55	21
40–49	16	12
50–59	5	5
≥60	1	0
Totals	156	57

*Age distribution of 213 patients as it relates to their diagnosis of either internal derangement or degenerative joint disease.

OUR EXPERIENCE WITH ARTHROSCOPIC LYSIS AND LAVAGE

From the beginning of 1985 until the middle of 1989 we performed 340 arthroscopic procedures on 213 patients who had painful TMJ hypomobility. The youngest patient was 10 years old and the oldest was 60 years old. The average age was 30 years (Table 5–1). There were 198 female patients and 15 male patients. The average duration of symptoms prior to the arthroscopic procedure was 3 years and 2 months. There were 127 bilateral procedures and 86 unilateral procedures performed.

Of the 340 arthroscopic procedures, 34 were diagnostic only. Three hundred six were therapeutic (i.e., surgical or operative) as well. All 34 diagnostic arthroscopies involved immediate arthrotomies. Most of the arthrotomies were performed on patients who were under 40 years of age.

The preoperative diagnosis of 156 of the 213 patients (73%) was internal derangement with persistent closed-lock. Fifty-seven of the patients (27%) had a preoperative diagnosis of degenerative joint disease (osteoarthritis) (Table 5–2).

RESULTS OF ARTHROSCOPIC LYSIS AND LAVAGE

A retrospective evaluation of these patients was carried out by means of periodic clinical examinations and chart reviews. A successful result was characterized by increased mandibular opening, mobility, and function and by decreased pain and disability. Results were classified as excellent, good, or poor. An excellent result was defined as an interincisal opening of 40 mm or greater (or an opening 3 fingers in breadth) causing minimum or no pain, minimum dietary and functional restrictions, and no sense of disability. A good result was defined as an opening of 30–35 mm (or an opening 2½ fingers in breadth) causing minimum to moderate pain, moderate dietary and functional restrictions, and a minimum to moderate sense of disability. A poor result was characterized by an opening of less than 30 mm (or an opening less than 2 fingers in breadth) causing significant pain, significant dietary and functional restrictions, and a sense of major disability.

One hundred ninety-two of the 221 joints with closed-lock (86.9%) had an excellent result following arthroscopic lysis and lavage. Twenty-one (9.5%) had a good result. Eight (3.6%) had a poor result. Seventy-two of the 85 joints with degenerative joint disease

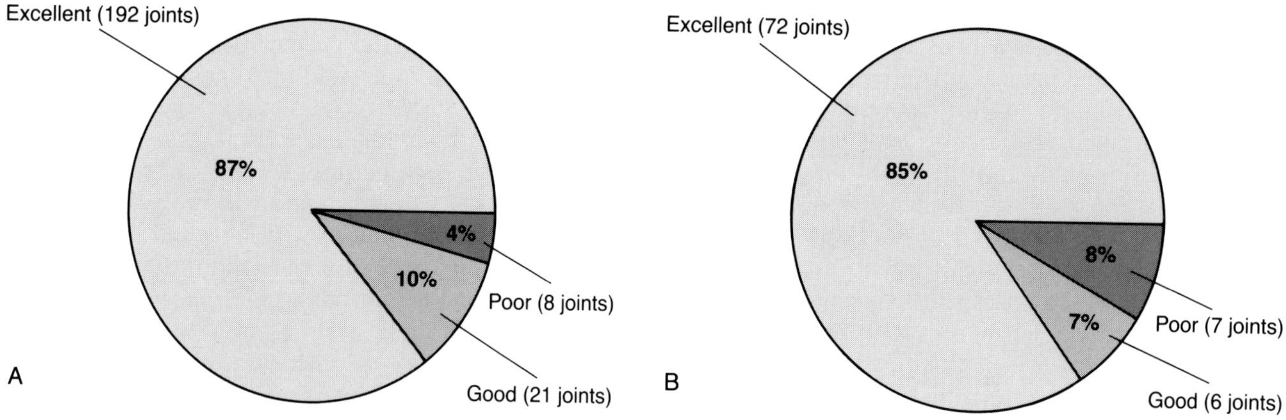

FIGURE 5–1. Postoperative results of arthroscopic lysis and lavage. *A*—Treatment outcome in patients with a preoperative diagnosis of internal derangement (221 joints). *B*—Treatment outcome in patients with a preoperative diagnosis of degenerative joint disease (85 joints).

TABLE 5–3. RESULTS OF ARTHROSCOPIC LYSIS AND LAVAGE BY YEAR*

Year	Number of Patients	Number of Excellent Results (%)	Number of Good Results (%)	Number of Poor Results (%)
1985	34	26 (76%)	4 (12%)	4 (12%)
1986	69	56 (81%)	10 (14%)	3 (4%)
1987	79	73 (92%)	3 (4%)	3 (4%)
1988	70	63 (90%)	6 (9%)	1 (1%)
1989	54	46 (85%)	5 (9%)	3 (6%)
Totals	306	264 (86%)	28 (9%)	14 (5%)

*Distribution of postoperative results (rated as excellent, good or poor) by the year of surgery from 1985 to 1989.

(84.7%) had an excellent result, 7 (8.2%) had a good result, and 6 (7.1%) had a poor result (Fig. 5–1). Yearly results were also evaluated (Table 5–3).

FAILURES OF LYSIS AND LAVAGE

In total, 14 of the 306 joints (4.5%) that underwent arthroscopic lysis and lavage failed. Factors that likely influenced failure included uncontrolled bruxism (6 joints), disk perforations and advanced osseous pathology (4 joints), systemic arthritis (3 joints), and previous arthrotomy (1 joint).

All 6 patients with joints with uncontrolled bruxism had continuous physical therapy and counseling to eliminate parafunctional muscle activity. Four had subsequent arthrotomies with disk removal followed by Silastic implants. One hundred per cent of these procedures failed. Two joints were treated nonsurgically after failed arthroscopy but continued to do poorly.

RESULTS OF ARTHROSCOPIC LYSIS AND LAVAGE IN THE TREATMENT OF DISK PERFORATIONS

Seventeen of the joints undergoing arthroscopy had large disk perforations. Three of the 17 joints underwent immediate arthrotomy, and all 3 of these joints underwent diskectomy. There were 2 excellent results and 1 good result after diskectomy. The other 14 joints with large perforations were treated with arthroscopic lysis and lavage. The results are presented in Table 5–4.

RESULTS OF ARTHROSCOPIC LYSIS AND LAVAGE IN THE TREATMENT OF PAINFUL JOINTS AFTER PREVIOUS ARTHROTOMY (EXCLUDING IMPLANTS)

In our series, there were 26 joints with painful status after arthrotomy. Twenty-two joints underwent disk repair procedures, and 4 underwent only diskectomy. Patients with implants were not placed in this category. All 26 joints underwent arthroscopic lysis and lavage to treat painful hypomobility. Nineteen of the 22 joints undergoing disk repair had an excellent result, 2 had a good result, and 1 had a poor result. Two of the 4 joints undergoing diskectomy had excellent results, 2 had good results, and none had a poor result (Table 5–5).

RESULTS OF ARTHROSCOPIC LYSIS AND LAVAGE IN THE TREATMENT OF PAINFUL JOINT HYPOMOBILITY STATUS AFTER MANDIBULAR SAGITTAL OSTEOTOMIES

TMJ internal derangement resulting in pain and mandibular hypomobility status after mandibular sagittal osteotomy has been reported by several authors. Sanders and colleagues[19] have treated 15 female patients with this problem. Thirteen of these patients had bilateral TMJ problems, and 2 had unilateral joint problems. All patients had mandibular advancement for retrognathia. None of the patients had significant

TABLE 5–4. RESULTS OF ARTHROSCOPIC LYSIS AND LAVAGE*

Result	Number of Patients (%)
Excellent	10 (71)
Good	0 (0)
Poor	4 (29)
Total	14 (100)

*Results of lysis and lavage in 14 patients who had arthroscopically observed disk perforations.

TABLE 5–5. RESULTS OF ARTHROSCOPIC LYSIS AND LAVAGE AFTER ARTHROTOMY

Painful Joints After a Previous Arthrotomic Procedure		Results of Lysis and Lavage (Number of Joints)		
Procedure	Number of Joints	Excellent	Good	Poor
Disk Repair	22	19	2	1
Diskectomy	4	2	2	0

TABLE 5–6. ARTHROSCOPIC FINDINGS IN 28 PAINFUL HYPOMOBILE JOINTS AFTER MANDIBULAR SAGITTAL OSTEOTOMY

Finding	Number of Joints
Displaced Disk	26
Morphologic Changes	26
Adhesions	26
Synovitis	20
Perforated or Destroyed Disk	6
Eburnation	2

preoperative TMJ symptoms. Postoperatively, all had preauricular pain, mandibular hypomobility, and joint crepitus. Postoperative arthroscopic findings are presented in Table 5–6. The duration of symptoms was 5 months to 2 years 7 months, with an average of 1 year 3 months.

Eight of the 28 involved joints (29%) had evidence of closed-lock, 14 (50%) had closed-lock with early degenerative joint disease, and 6 (21%) had advanced degenerative disease. The average opening before arthroscopy was 27 mm with a range of 16–39 mm.

All 15 patients (28 joints) underwent arthroscopic lysis and lavage as an outpatient hospital procedure. There were no complications, and all patients had postoperative physical therapy. The range of clinical follow-up was from 6 months to 4 years. The average postarthroscopic interincisal opening was 38 mm with a range of 34–42 mm. The average improvement of opening was 11 mm, with a range of 2–18 mm (Table 5–7). There was significant pain level reduction in all of the patients.

TABLE 5–7. IMPROVEMENT IN OPENING BEFORE AND AFTER ARTHROSCOPIC LYSIS AND LAVAGE FOLLOWING MANDIBULAR SAGITTAL OSTEOTOMY (15 PATIENTS)

Patient	Preoperative Opening (mm)	Postoperative Opening (mm)	Improvement (mm)
1	25	35	10
2	29	35	6
3	27	35	8
4	39	41	2
5	39	42	3
6	23	35	12
7	16	34	18
8	30	40	10
9	26	36	10
10	31	40	9
11	26	38	12
12	20	35	15
13	22	38	16
14	26	42	16
15	23	37	14

SUMMARY

Arthroscopic lysis and lavage is a procedure that has been advocated for approximately 5 years. It has been proven to be an effective operative arthroscopic procedure. It is especially effective in treating patients with painful TMJ hypomobility secondary to closed-lock and degenerative joint disease. The results presented here have been confirmed by other investigators.[8,14–16]

REFERENCES

1. Sanders, B. Arthroscopic surgery of the temporomandibular joint: Treatment of internal derangement with persistent closed lock. Oral Surg (1986), 62:361.
2. Sanders, B. Arthroscopy of the temporomandibular joint. Richard Wolf Medical Instruments Corp. (1987).
3. Sanders, B; Buoncristiani, R. Diagnostic and surgical arthroscopy of the temporomandibular joint: Clinical experience with 137 procedures over a 2-year period. J Craniomandib Dis Fac Oral Pain (1987), 1:202.
4. Sanders, B; Murakami, K; Clark, G. Diagnostic and Surgical Arthroscopy of the Temporomandibular Joint. Philadelphia, W. B. Saunders Co. (1989).
5. Merrill, R. Personal communication, 1989.
6. Schwartz, R. Personal communication, 1989.
7. Davis, C; Kaminishi, R. Personal communication, 1989.
8. Indresano, T. Personal communication, 1989.
9. Dolwick, F. Personal communication, 1989.
10. Murakami, K. Personal communication, 1989.
11. Van Sickels, J. Personal communication, 1989.
12. Sanders, B. TMJ lysis and lavage: A 5-year experience. Lecture presented at the Fourth International Symposium on Arthroscopy for TMJ Disorders, Maui, Hawaii, December 1989.
13. White, D. Arthroscopic Surgery. Abstract presented at the Third International Symposium on Arthroscopy for TMJ Disorders, New York, New York, December 1988.
14. Moore, L. Arthroscopic Surgery for Treatment of Restrictive Temporomandibular Joint Disease: A Prospective Longitudinal Study (abstract). Fourth International Symposium on Arthroscopy for TMJ Disorders, Maui, Hawaii, December 1989.
15. Indresano, T. Arthroscopic surgery of the temporomandibular joint: Report of 64 patients with long-term follow-up. J Oral Maxillofac Surg (1989), 47:439–441.
16. Montgomery, M; et al. Arthroscopic surgery: Effects on signs, symptoms, and disk position. J Oral and Maxillofac Surg (1989), 47:1263–1271.
17. Dolwick, F. Comparison of TMJ arthroscopy and arthrotomy. Lecture presented at the Third International Symposium on Arthroscopy for TMJ Disorders, New York, New York, December 1988.
18. Porter, B; Zeitler, D. Comparison of TMJ arthroscopy and arthrotomy. Abstract presented at the Fourth International Symposium on Arthroscopy for TMJ Disorders, Maui, Hawaii, December 1989.
19. Sanders, B; Kaminishi, R; Buoncristiani, R; Davis, C. Arthroscopic surgery for treatment of temporomandibular joint hypomobility after mandibular sagittal osteotomy. Oral Surg Oral Med Oral Pathol. (In Press).

Six

Arthroscopic Surgery for the Treatment of Restrictive Temporomandibular Joint Disease
A Prospective Longitudinal Study

LARRY J. MOORE, D.D.S., M.S.

Arthroscopic surgery for the treatment of internal derangements of the temporomandibular joint (TMJ) has gained wide acceptance and popularity among oral and maxillofacial surgeons in the United States. Published reports of arthroscopic surgery indicate a short-term success rate of 85% or higher based largely on subjective criteria and retrospective analysis.[1-4] The long-term results of arthroscopic surgery based on objective criteria and prospective design are important to establish the technique as legitimate therapy.

A prospective longitudinal study was designed in order to evaluate the efficacy of arthroscopic surgery of the TMJ for treatment of restrictive TMJ disease. For the purposes of this study, restrictive TMJ disease is defined as painful limitation of mandibular range of motion, arising from documented internal derangement of the TMJ, using either magnetic resonance imaging (MRI) or arthrotomography. Using the arthroscopic staging system proposed by Bronstein, patients included in this study were judged to have stage III or IV disease preoperatively.[5]

MATERIALS AND METHODS

Sixty-three consecutive patients ranging in age from 17 to 68 years were admitted to the study over a 3-year period. The average age of these patients was 34.7 years; 92% were female, 8% male (Fig. 6-1). All patients presented with complaints of limited mandibular opening and pain that had been refractory to nonsurgical therapy. None had received previous surgery of the TMJ. Nonsurgical therapy consisted of behavior modification, nonsteroidal antiinflammatory drugs, occlusal appliances, and physical therapy in all cases. The average duration of nonsurgical therapy prior to surgery was 12.2 months, with a range of eight weeks to eight years. The average duration of painful symptoms prior to the initial interview was 31.4 months, with a range of 1 week to 13 years.

All patients were interviewed by the author and asked to complete questionnaires preoperatively and at regular intervals postoperatively. Postoperative interviews were recorded at 4, 8, and 12 weeks after surgery, then every 3 months until 1 year after surgery, and thereafter every 6 months for the duration of the study. Patients were asked to rank their pain on subjective analog scales of 0 to 10, where 0 was no pain, and 10 represented the patients' worst pain experience. A similar analog scale was used to rate the patients' subjective dysfunction; in this scale, zero represented the ability to chew normally, and 10 represented the complete inability to chew (liquid diet).

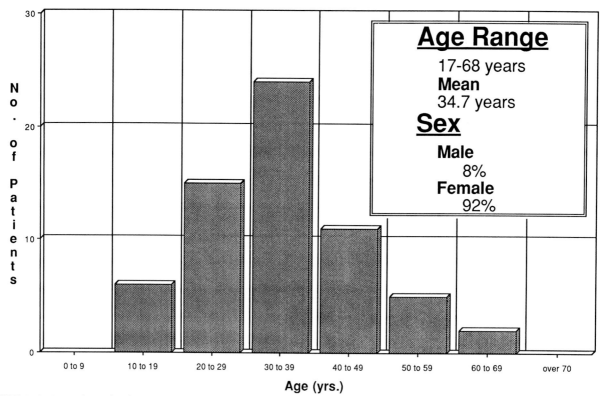

FIGURE 6–1. Age and sex distribution for the study group (n = 63). The great majority of patients were female (n = 58), and clustered around the fourth decade of life.

Objective measurements of mandibular range of motion were made with calipers and a millimeter ruler using passive assistance. The maximum interincisal opening (MIO), right and left lateral excursions, and protrusion were measured preoperatively and at regular intervals postoperatively.

Arthroscopic lysis and lavage, lateral capsular release, and motorized shaving were performed as needed on 120 TMJs in the 63 patients. All surgeries were performed by the author in an outpatient hospital setting. Patients underwent 3 to 8 weeks of postoperative physical therapy to normalize and maintain range of motion. A full liquid diet was prescribed for the first two weeks postoperatively, then two weeks of soft foods, followed by the careful return to a normal diet as tolerated.

Mean follow-up time for the study group was 52 months, with a range of 36 to 75 months. Statistical analysis was performed using a Student's t-test to compare the preoperative values for pain, dysfunction, and range of motion with those seen at 1 year, 2 years, 3 years, and 4 years postoperatively (Tables 6–1 and 6–2). Clinical success was determined by statistically significant improvement in all three criteria ($p<.05$). Patients failing to show significant improvement in any one category were classified as treatment failures. These patients were followed for 1 year before additional surgical therapy was offered.

RESULTS

Mandibular range of motion improved rapidly following arthroscopic surgery, stabilizing at about 8 to

TABLE 6–1. OBJECTIVE CRITERIA*

$\bar{x} \pm sd$	Preoperative (63)	1 Year Postoperative (63)	2 Years Postoperative (58)	3 Years Postoperative (57)	4 Years Postoperative (28)
Maximum interincisal opening	28.5 ± 6.3 mm	40.3 ± 4.2 mm	40.7 ± 2.2 mm	40.2 ± 2.8 mm	41.0 ± 2.3 mm
Right lateral excursion	3.5 ± 2.14 mm	8.6 ± 1.9 mm	8.4 ± 2.2 mm	8.5 ± 2.0 mm	8.9 ± 1.7 mm
Left lateral excursion	4.2 ± 2.9 mm	8.8 ± 2.0 mm	8.6 ± 1.8 mm	8.6 ± 1.7 mm	8.7 ± 1.4 mm
Protrusion	3.0 ± 2.5 mm	7.4 ± 1.8 mm	7.2 ± 2.3 mm	7.2 ± 1.9 mm	7.5 ± 1.5 mm

*Mean values for range of motion measurements are shown plus or minus one standard deviation. All postoperative values at 1, 2, 3, and 4 years are significantly greater than the respective preoperative values ($p < .05$).

TABLE 6–2. SUBJECTIVE CRITERIA*

Analog Scale 0 to 10 $\bar{x}$ ± sd	Preoperative (63)	1 Year Postoperative (63)	2 Years Postoperative (58)	3 Years Postoperative (57)	4 Years Postoperative (28)
Subjective pain	8.2 ± 1.5	1.5 ± 1.7	1.1 ± 1.3	0.82 ± 1.0	0.8 ± 1.2
Subjective dysfunction	7.1 ± 1.4	3.1 ± 1.6	2.3 ± 1.4	2.2 ± 1.2	2.0 ± 1.0

*Mean values for subjective pain and dysfunction are shown plus or minus one standard deviation. All postoperative values at 1, 2, 3, and 4 years are significantly greater than the respective preoperative values.

10 weeks postoperatively (Figs. 6–2 and 6–3). Mean preoperative and postoperative values for mandibular range of motion are listed in Table 6–1. The postoperative values listed are all significantly greater than the respective preoperative values (p<.05). The average net increase in MIO was 12 mm following arthroscopic surgery. The average net increase was 5.1 mm for right lateral excursion, 4.5 mm for left lateral excursion, and 4.3 mm for protrusion.

Subjective pain scores dropped rapidly following arthroscopic surgery (Fig. 6–4), with many patients reporting greatly reduced pain as early as one week after surgery. Pain scores showed the greatest interval improvement at the 4-week postoperative interview, then improved more gradually until 6 months after surgery.

Subjective dysfunction scores improved less rapidly than pain scores (Fig. 6–5). The 4-week postoperative scores are of limited value, since many patients were still on a restricted diet at that point; however, steady improvement was noted, stabilizing at 6 months.

The mean postoperative pain and dysfunction scores are significantly lower than the preoperative values at 1, 2, 3, and 4 years postoperatively (Table 6–2). The average net decrease in pain scores was 7.1 points, and the average net decrease in dysfunction scores was 4.7 points. The improvement in both pain and dysfunction scores is statistically significant (p<.05).

Of the 63 patients accepted into the study protocol, 55 (87%) had successful results at 1 year according to the criteria described earlier. Eight patients failed to show significant improvement in at least one category, and 5 of these elected to have a second surgical procedure after 1 year. These patients were dropped from the study after the 1-year interview. At 2 years after surgery 87% remained successful outcomes. One patient with a successful outcome reinjured her TMJ in a motor vehicle accident 2 years and 3 months after surgery and was dropped from the study. At 4 years after surgery no additional treatment failures were seen. Between 4 and 6 years, 2 patients were lost to follow-up, but no additional failures were seen. All of

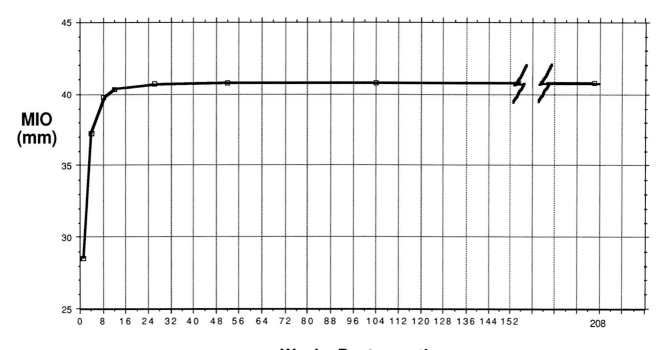

Weeks Postoperative

FIGURE 6–2. Maximum interincisal opening (MIO) versus time. Rapid improvement was seen from a mean of 28.5 mm preoperatively to slightly over 40 mm at 12 weeks postoperatively. This change remained stable throughout the follow-up period.

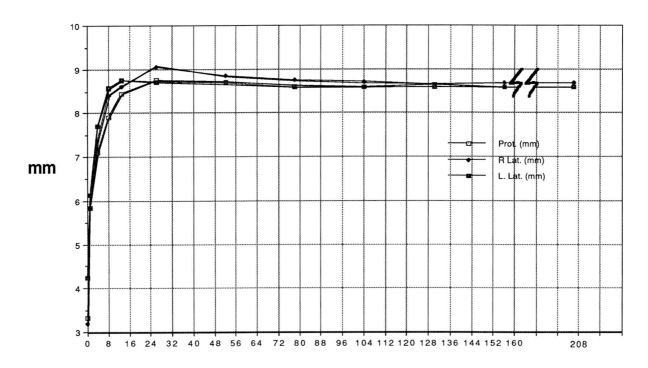

Weeks Postoperative

FIGURE 6–3. Rapid improvement was observed in right and left lateral excursions, and protrusion was seen in the first 12 weeks postoperatively. These changes remained stable throughout the follow-up period (*open squares*: protrusion; *solid diamonds*: right lateral excursion; *solid squares*: left lateral excursion).

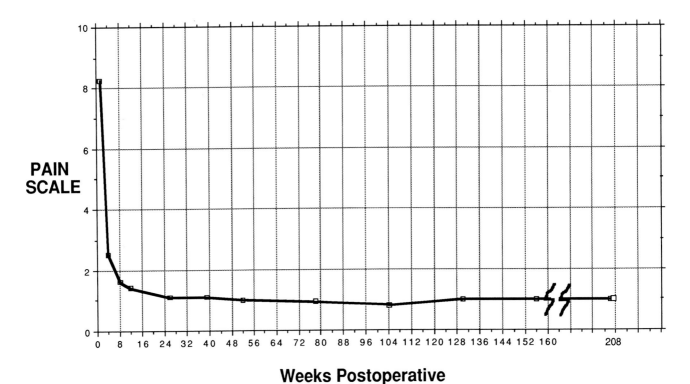

Weeks Postoperative

FIGURE 6–4. Subjective pain scores showed the greatest interval change in the first four weeks after arthroscopic surgery. No significant change occurred after three months postoperatively.

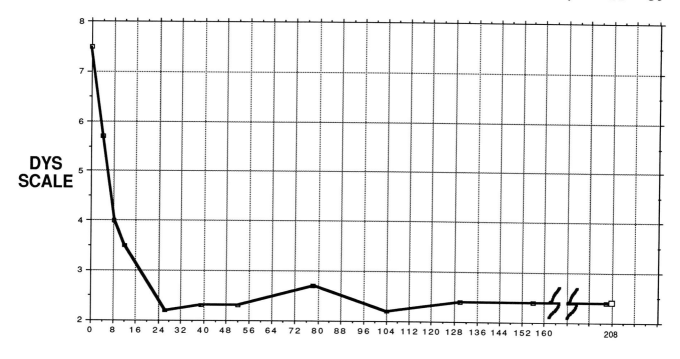

Weeks Postoperative

FIGURE 6–5. Subjective dysfunction scores show the greatest interval change in the period from 4 weeks to 8 weeks postoperatively. The initial rate of improvement for dysfunction scores was slower than for pain scores, and the level at which dysfunction scores stabilized was higher than that for pain scores (approximately 2.4 versus 1.1).

the treatment failures occurred within 6 months of surgery, and outcome did not significantly improve with continued nonsurgical therapy.

A comparison of the 8 patients failing to improve after arthroscopic surgery with the study group as a whole revealed no significant differences in age, sex, or duration of symptoms. A review of the findings at surgery (Table 6–3) showed the failure group more likely to have disk perforation and degenerative joint disease than the study group as a whole. Although 8% of the disks were perforated in the study group, 50% of the failures showed disk perforation. Degenerative bony changes were noted in 15% of the study group and in 75% of the failures. These differences were not found to be statistically significant.

TABLE 6–3. FINDINGS AT SURGERY*

Pathology	Percent	Number of Joints
Synovitis	96.0	117
Anterior disk position	92.0	115
Fibrous adhesions	58.0	71
Altered disk morphology	35.0	59
Fibrosynovial adhesions	33.0	40
Degenerative joint disease	15.0	18
Perforation	8.0	10

*Findings at surgery are shown based on the number of joints exhibiting arthroscopic evidence of the pathology listed.

DISCUSSION

This study was designed to test the efficacy of arthroscopic surgery for the treatment of restrictive TMJ disease manifested as painful restriction of mandibular motion arising from internal derangement. The important questions addressed by this study are whether statistically significant changes in objective measurements (range of motion) and subjective measurements (pain and dysfunction) occur after arthroscopic surgery.

It is clear that significant improvement in range of motion did occur in 87% of the patients in the study and that this improvement is stable for at least 4 years at confidence levels of $p < .05$. Likewise, pain and dysfunction scores showed significant improvement after arthroscopic surgery, and remained stable for at least 4 years at confidence levels of $p < .05$. Patients in the study group who had been followed for 5 or 6 years showed similar stable results although the numbers were too small to permit statistical correlation.

As mentioned previously, all treatment failures occurred within the first 6 months after surgery. Patients in this group were judged to have had stage IV or V disease using the criteria described by Bronstein. This finding is not statistically significant, but it seems likely that patients failing arthroscopic surgery in this study were more likely to have more advanced internal derangement and more severe degenerative joint disease than those who had clinically successful outcomes.

CONCLUSIONS

Eighty-seven percent of the 63 patients presenting with restrictive TMJ disease showed statistically significant improvement in range of motion and reduction in pain and dysfunction after arthroscopic surgery. These results were stable over a 4-year follow-up period at confidence levels of $p<.05$. Patients failing to improve were identified within 6 months of surgery; these patients showed a tendency to have more severe internal derangements and a higher frequency of de-

generative joint disease than patients enjoying stable successful outcomes.

REFERENCES

1. Indresano, TA. Arthroscopic surgery of the temporomandibular joint: Report of 64 patients with long-term follow-up. J Oral Maxillofac Surg (1989), 47:439–441.
2. White, RD. Retrospective analysis of 100 consecutive surgical arthroscopies of the temporomandibular joint. J Oral Maxillofac Surg (1989), 47:1014–1021.
3. Moses, JJ; Poker, ID. TMJ Arthroscopic surgery: An analysis of 237 patients. J Oral Maxillofac Surg (1989), 47:790–794.
4. Sanders, B; Buoncristiani, R. Diagnostic and surgical arthroscopy of the temporomandibular joint: Clinical experience with 137 procedures over a two-year period. J Craniomandib Dis Fac Oral Pain (1987), 1:202–211.
5. Bronstein, SL. Diagnostic and operative arthroscopy: Historical perspectives and indications. Oral Maxillofac Surg Clin N Am (1989), 1:59–68.

Seven

Effectiveness of Arthroscopy
A Retrospective Study

EDWARD L. MOSBY, D.D.S., F.A.C.D.
BRETT L. FERGUSON, D.D.S.
BRUCE B. CHISHOLM, D.D.S.

Arthroscopic surgery of the temporomandibular joint (TMJ) has become an important and appropriate option in the treatment of TMJ dysfunction. There are multiple treatment modalities available to treat TMJ dysfunction, with TMJ surgery being a final option when indicated. The surgical modalities include arthroscopy and arthrotomy.

The historical perspectives of TMJ arthroscopy have been enumerated by various authors and summarized by Bronstein.[1] Arthroscopy was introduced in this country in the 1980s and has subsequently enjoyed a rapid development and an increase in popularity as it has filled the need for a less invasive surgical procedure. Initial reports have detailed the normal TMJ arthroscopic anatomy and diagnostic potential[2,3] as well as the therapeutic effect of the arthroscopic surgical procedure.[4-6]

The International Study Group for the Advancement of TMJ Arthroscopy has spearheaded the impetus for research, continuing education, and the development of guidelines for clinical privileges, and has provided a rationale for TMJ arthroscopy. A study prepared by the group was presented at the Fourth Annual Symposium on Arthroscopy of the Temporomandibular Joint in December 1989.

Nonsurgical therapy of the TMJ has not been replaced by arthroscopic surgery. Rather, TMJ arthroscopy serves as a minimally invasive surgical procedure in patients in whom nonsurgical methods, such as splint therapy, have not been successful.

The purpose of this study is to compare preoperative and postoperative signs and symptoms following TMJ arthroscopic surgery.

METHODS AND MATERIALS

This study included 43 patients who underwent a total of 53 TMJ arthroscopies after nonsurgical therapy failed to relieve symptoms to a manageable level. There were 32 women and 11 men receiving 11 bilateral procedures and 31 unilateral procedures. The arthroscopic procedure was each patient's first TMJ surgical procedure. All patients selected for this study were to have at least 6 months' postsurgical follow-up (Table 7–1).

Pre- and postoperative measurements included interincisal opening, lateral and protrusive excursions, headaches, and muscle and joint pain. Pain was graded from 0 to 10, with 10 being the most severe pain. All patients underwent lysis, lavage, and débridement of the superior joint space using a standard surgical approach (Fig. 7–1).

TABLE 7–1. COMPARISON OF THE NUMBER OF PATIENTS WITH THE NUMBER OF UNILATERAL AND BILATERAL ARTHROSCOPIC PROCEDURES

43 patients	53 arthroscopies
32 females	31 unilateral
11 males	11 bilateral

PRE-OPERATIVE NON-SURGICAL THERAPY
SUPERIOR JOINT ARTHROSCOPY

- **LYSIS**
- **LAVAGE**
- **DÉBRIDEMENT**
- **MOBILIZATION**

POST-OPERATIVE SPLINT

PHYSICAL THERAPY

FIGURE 7–1. Treatment regimen.

TABLE 7–3. DISTRIBUTION OF PRESURGICAL IMAGING*

Type of Imaging	Percent (n) of Patients
Panoramic imaging	93 (40)
Transcranial imaging	58 (25)
Magnetic resonance imaging	38 (16)
Tomograms	21 (9)
Arthrograms	9 (4)
Computed tomography scan	7 (3)

*Sixty-five percent (28) of the patients' presurgical images showed some degenerative changes in one or both joints.

The mean age for all patients was 33 years, with a range of 13–59 years (Table 7–2). Preoperatively 93% (40) of the patients had panoramic imaging performed, 58% (25) underwent transcranial imaging, 38% (16) underwent magnetic resonance imaging (MRI), 21% (9) tomography, 9% (4) arthrography, and 7% (3) underwent computed tomography (CT). Twenty-eight patients had radiographic evidence of degenerative joint disease (Table 7–3).

Preoperative diagnosis indicated 53% (23) with anterior disk displacement with reduction, 44% (19) with anterior disk displacement without reduction, 1.5% (1) with hemarthrosis, and 1.5% (1) with fibrous ankylosis (Fig. 7–2). Sixty-five per cent (28) were in class I occlusion, 19% (8) were in class II, and 9% (4) were class III (Table 7–4). Eighty-one per cent (35) of the patients had pain preoperatively for greater than 6 months.

RESULTS

Range of Motion

The resulting data showed an increase in interincisal opening, as well as an increase in lateral and protrusive movements. Preoperatively, 71% (31) of the patients had an interincisal opening of less than 30 mm. Postoperatively, 65% (28) had an interincisal opening of greater than 40 mm. Similarly, patients exhibited an increase in both lateral and protrusive excursions. Preoperatively, 58% (25) had a lateral excursion of 7–10 mm, while 79% (34) had the same range postoper-

atively. Forty-seven per cent (20) of the patients had a preoperative protrusive excursion of less than 7 mm, and 79% (34) had a postoperative protrusive excursion of 7–10 mm (Fig. 7–3).

Pain

Pain generally decreased in all patients. A decrease in pain to 2 or less on a scale of 0–10 was observed in 88% (36) of the patients. Preoperatively, 69% (30) of the patients had pain subjectively described as between 9 and 10, with 10 being the most severe pain. Furthermore, 90% (39) described their pain as greater than or equal to 7. Postoperatively, 88% (38) of the patients described their pain as being less than or equal to 2 after 1 month, 91% (39) after 6 months, and 86% (30) of the 35 patients in the follow-up period described their pain as at this level after 1–3 years. Patients with greater than 3 years' follow-up were not considered statistically significant because of their small number (5) (Table 7–5). Patients stated that their pain was disruptive to their lifestyles when it was reported to be 6 or greater on the 1 to 10 scale.

Headaches

Seventy-nine per cent (34) of the patients reported that they had headaches prior to arthroscopy, and only

TABLE 7–2. DISTRIBUTION OF PATIENTS BY AGE

Age (in years)	Number of Patients	Age (in years)	Number of Patients
10–14	1	35–39	7
15–19	7	40–44	5
20–24	6	45–49	1
25–29	7	50–55	1
30–34	8		
Average age			29.5
Mean age			33.0

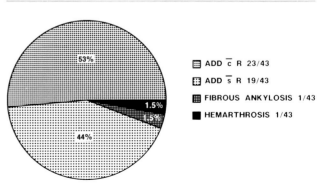

FIGURE 7–2. Number of patients in each joint disorder or diagnostic group (ADD: anterior disk displacement; R: reduction).

TABLE 7–4. DISTRIBUTION OF PATIENTS ACCORDING TO CLASSIFICATION OF OCCLUSION, AND NUMBER OF PATIENTS HAVING OCCLUSION-ALTERING TREATMENT BEFORE ARTHROSCOPY

	Occlusion	Number of Patients*
Edentulous 1	Class I	28
Open-bite 1	Class II	8
Mutilated 1	Class III	4

*Number of patients having previous orthodontic treatment = 10; number of patients having previous orthognathic surgery = 1.

19% (8) stated they had headaches at their most recent postarthroscopic evaluation. Two of these patients had persistent migraine-type headaches (Table 7–6).

Muscle Tenderness

Prior to arthroscopy, fewer than 50% of the patients who underwent arthroscopy had muscle tenderness in response to palpation of one or more of the six muscles chosen (unilateral or bilateral was counted as 1 patient). No more than 7% (3) of the patients had tenderness in one or more of the muscles subsequent to arthroscopy (Table 7–7).

Joint Noise

Joint noises are not reported in this study, as many of the patients displayed such noises after arthroscopy. The noises may or may not have changed in character from the prearthroscopic joint noises. Whether the patients do or do not have postsurgical joint noises does not appear to be relevant to the successful reduction of pain or to an increase in the range of motion.

Symptoms

A review of the histories revealed that 84% (36) of the patients had symptoms of 6 years' duration or less. Thirty-seven per cent (16) had symptoms for less than

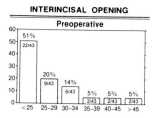
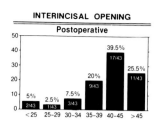
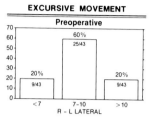
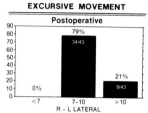
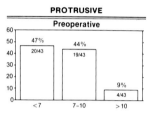
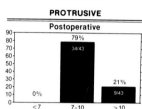

FIGURE 7–3. Range of motion: Vertical opening and lateral and protrusive excursions in patients before and after arthroscopy (in millimeters). The postoperative measurements reported were recorded at the patients' last postsurgical visits, i.e., six patients with a 6-month to 1-year follow-up, 35 with a 1- to 3-year follow-up, and five with a greater than 3-year follow-up.

1 year, 23% (10) for 1–2 years, 23% (10) for 3–6 years, 12% (5) for 7–10 years, and 4% (2) for 11–20 years.

The most frequently reported cause of symptoms was a motor vehicle accident (33%). The remaining causes in descending order were unknown (21%), work-related injury (14%), dental treatment (12%), assault (9%), fall (5%), medical treatment (5%), and sports injury (2%) (Table 7–8).

Previous Therapy

A total of 79% (34) of the patients had previously received nonsurgical therapy by two or more practi-

TABLE 7–5. DISTRIBUTION OF PATIENTS REPORTING PAIN OF VARYING LEVELS OF INTENSITY BEFORE ARTHROSCOPY AND AT THE INTERVALS INDICATED AFTER ARTHROSCOPY

Pain Intensity (1–10)	Before Arthroscopy n (%)	1 Month n (%)	6 Months n (%)	1–3 Years n (%)	>3 Years n (%)
0–2	0 (0)	38 (88)	39 (91)	30 (86)	5 (100)
3–4	2 (5)	2 (5)	1 (2)	2 (6)	0 (0)
5–6	2 (5)	0 (0)	1 (2)	2 (6)	0 (0)
7–8	9 (21)	2 (5)	2 (5)	1 (3)	0 (0)
9–10	30 (69)	1 (2)	0 (0)	0 (0)	0 (0)
Total	43	43	43	35	5

TABLE 7–6. DISTRIBUTION OF PATIENTS REPORTING HEADACHES BEFORE AND AFTER ARTHROSCOPY

Frequency of Headaches	Number of Patients	
	Before Arthroscopy	*After Arthroscopy*
None	9	35
<3 per week	3	3
3–5 per week	7	0
Daily	22	3
Migraine	2	2

tioners, and 28% (12) had been treated by at least five practitioners (Table 7–9). The treatments rendered in order of frequency were medication (95%), splints (all types) (65%), occlusal equilibration (32%), physical therapy (26%), orthodontics (23%), and psychologic counseling (12%). Thirty-five per cent (15) of the patients reported having received only one therapeutic modality, 26% (11) received two modalities, 32% (14) received three modalities, and 5% (2) received four, five, and six different treatment modalities (Table 7–10).

DISCUSSION

The surgical treatment of disorders of the TMJ has always been directed at the restoration of normal biologic form and functional anatomy. Surgery is followed by a recuperative period including vigorous physical therapy directed toward the return of the TMJ to within normal functional range and painless function or toward a reduction in pain and an increase in function that is manageable for the patient. This study shows that success is attainable regardless of the postsurgical position of the disk, as success was judged based not on a reduction in joint noise during function, but rather on the relief of pain and a return to the normal limits of range of motion. Numerous retrospective studies, including our studies at the University of Missouri–Kansas City, have changed many sur-

geons' beliefs regarding the importance of disk position in obtaining a successful surgical result.[7–13] This does not mean that we forget the importance of a normal disk-condyle-fossa functional relationship. However, we need to maintain this relationship in proper perspective. Attempts by expert arthroscopists to find a way to reposition the normal disk should be applauded, not abandoned.

Surgical procedures to reestablish a normal structural relationship should continue to serve as treatment options when appropriate. Arthroscopy with lysis, lavage, débridement, and mobilization has been shown in short-term retrospective studies to be a viable treatment option. At this time, we are not totally aware of which patients with which types of internal derangements will benefit the most from lysis, lavage, débridement, and mobilization. To date, none of the patients in this study has required a second surgical procedure, whether arthroscopic or open. It is conceivable that there are patients who will require re-arthroscopy or open joint surgery should their pain or dysfunction again increase to a level that is not manageable for them. If some patients who have had lysis, lavage, débridement, and mobilization show deterioration and need additional surgical procedures, does this mean that the arthroscopic procedures were failures? A more realistic view would be that the management of organic joint disease is a continuum of nonsurgical and surgical management.

Many people have a functional occlusion and a normal or functional range of motion, yet have an internal derangement in one or both of their TMJs. Should not success then be gauged based on the reduction of pain to a level that is manageable and on the return to a functional range of motion?

In the group of patients in this study bilateral arthroscopic procedures were not the norm. Only 25% (11) of the patients underwent bilateral procedures. Our criterion used in determining bilateralism was the patients' perception of their pain or dysfunction, not organic joint disease or the type of internal derangement. If a patient had documented joint disease or

TABLE 7–7. RESPONSE TO PALPATION OF THE MUSCLES OF MASTICATION, THE NECK, AND THE UPPER BACK BEFORE AND AFTER ARTHROSCOPY

Muscle	Pain Level* Before Arthroscopy				Pain Level* After Arthroscopy			
	0	*1*	*2*	*3*	*0*	*1*	*2*	*3*
Temporalis	28	8	6	1	41	2	0	0
Masseter	23	10	9	1	40	3	0	0
Sternocleidomastoid	27	9	6	1	43	0	0	0
Digastric	36	5	2	0	43	0	0	0
Trapezius	22	13	6	2	41	2	0	0
Splenius	25	12	4	2	41	2	0	0

*0 = no response; 1 = mildly painful; 2 = moderately painful; 3 = severely painful (patient retracted).

TABLE 7–8. CHRONICITY AND REPORTED ETIOLOGY OF SYMPTOMS

Chronicity of Symptoms	Number of Patients	Reported Etiology of Symptoms	Number of Patients
1 year	16	Motor vehicle accident	14
1–2 years	10	Unknown	9
3–6 years	10	Work-related injury	8
7–10 years	5	Dental treatment	5
11–15 years	1	Assault	4
16–20 years	1	Fall	2
		Medical treatment	2
		Sports injury	1

internal derangement on both sides, but his or her pain or dysfunction was disruptive on only one side, a unilateral procedure was selected.

SUMMARY

The results of this study show a definite improvement in mobility and reduction of pain following arthroscopic surgery of the TMJ. The beneficial results are most apparent in the generalized pain reduction and the increase in the range of motion.

There were 43 patients (32 women and 11 men) and 53 joints reviewed. Preoperative imaging studies included panoramic imaging (40), transcranial imaging (25), tomography (9), arthrography (4), CT (3), and MRI (16). Preoperative diagnoses included anterior displaced disk with reduction (23/43, or 53%), anterior displaced disk without reduction (19/43, or 44%), fibrous ankylosis (1/43, or 1.5%), and hemarthrosis (1/43, or 1.5%).

The majority of patients described their level of pain preoperatively as being greater than 7. Postoperatively, all but 1 patient described the level of pain as being less than 7. Ninety-three per cent had pain reduction to a level described as manageable, and 88% had reduction of their pain to a level of 2 or less on a scale of 0–10.

Patients who were deemed candidates for arthro-scopic surgery had in general undergone extensive nonsurgical therapy without success. Patients voiced their chief complaint as being debilitating pain that interfered with their daily lifestyle. Based on the findings in this study, patients with anterior disk displacement with or without reduction can benefit from the results of lysis, lavage, débridement, and mobilization of the TMJ and disk using arthroscopic procedures.

Increased mobility is another beneficial result of arthroscopic surgery of the TMJ. Preoperatively, the majority of patients had an interincisal opening of less than 25 mm, but postoperatively, the majority had an interincisal opening of greater than 40 mm. Patients were instructed preoperatively and postoperatively regarding an aggressive physical therapy program.

The results of this study are encouraging in the short term. Patients experience the relief of symptoms and are able to avoid more extensively invasive procedures. The results of this study concur with other current, short-term follow-ups. Long-term follow-ups will be necessary to see whether the actual and the short-term results obtained from arthroscopic surgery will endure. Arthroscopic surgery of the TMJ is a viable option in the selection of treatment for TMJ dysfunctions.

TABLE 7–9. PREVIOUS TREATMENT

Practitioners*	Patients†
0	1
1	8
2	10
3	6
4	6
5+	12

*Number of practitioners providing previous treatment.
†Number of patients receiving previous treatment from the indicated number of practitioners.

TABLE 7–10. NONSURGICAL TREATMENT BEFORE ARTHROSCOPY

Treatment	Number of Patients
Medication	41
Splints	28
Occlusal equilibration	14
Physical therapy	11
Orthodontics	10
Psychologic counseling	5
Number of Different Treatments	**Number of Patients**
1	15
2	11
3	14
4	2
5	2
6	2

REFERENCES

1. Bronstein, SL. Diagnostic and operative arthroscopy: Historic perspective and indications. Oral Maxillofac Surg Clin N Am (1989), 1:59.
2. Heffez, L; Blaustein, D. Diagnostic Arthroscopy of the temporomandibular joint: I. Normal arthroscopic findings. Oral Surg Oral Med Oral Pathol (1987), 64:653.
3. Blaustein, D; Heffez, L. Diagnostic arthroscopy of the temporomandibular joint. II. Arthroscopic findings of arthrographically diagnosed disc displacements. Oral Surg Oral Med Oral Pathol (1988), 65:135.
4. McCain, JP. Proceedings of the Abstract Sessions, American Association of Oral and Maxillofacial Surgeons Annual Meeting. Washington, DC. September 1985.
5. Sanders, B. Arthroscopic surgery of the temporomandibular joint: Treatment of internal derangements with persistent closed lock. Oral Surg Oral Med Oral Pathol (1986), 62:361.
6. Sanders, B. Diagnostic and surgical arthroscopy of the temporomandibular joint: Clinical experience with 137 procedures over a 2-year period. J Craniomandib Dis Fac Oral Pain (1987), 1:202.
7. Montgomery, MT; Van Sickles, JE; Harms, SE; Thrash, WJ. Arthroscopic TMJ surgery: Effects on signs, symptoms, and disc position. J Oral Maxillofac Surg (1989), 47:1263.
8. Moses, JJ; Sartoris, D; Glass, R; et al. The effect of arthroscopic surgical lysis and lavage of the superior joint space on TMJ disc position and mobility. J Oral Maxillofac Surg (1989), 47:674.
9. Indresano, AT. Arthroscopic surgery of the temporomandibular joint: Report of 64 patients with long-term follow-up. J Oral Maxillofac Surg (1989), 47:439.
10. White, RD. Retrospective analysis of 100 consecutive surgical arthroscopies of the temporomandibular joint. J Oral Maxillofac Surg (1989), 47:1014.
11. Israel, HA; Roser, SM. Patient response to temporomandibular joint arthroscopy: Preliminary findings in 24 patients. J Oral Maxillofac Surg (1989), 47:570.
12. Moses, JJ; Poker, ID. TMJ arthroscopic surgery: An analysis of 237 patients. J Oral Maxillofac Surg (1989), 47:790.
13. Gabler, MJ; Greene, CS; Palacios, E; Perry, HT. Effect of arthroscopic temporomandibular joint surgery on articular disk position. J Craniomandib Dis Fac Oral Pain (1989), 3:191.

Eight

A Retrospective Study Comparing Arthroscopic Surgery with Arthrotomy and Disk Repositioning

DEBORAH L. ZEITLER, D.D.S., M.S.
BRADLEY T. PORTER, D.D.S., M.S.

Surgical treatments for temporomandibular joint (TMJ) disorders have ranged from joint lavage to total joint replacement, from condylectomy to diskectomy, and from disk repair to disk mobilization. The choice of surgical treatment is generally made by the individual surgeon based on his or her experience, training, expertise, and clinical judgment. As the etiology and pathogenesis of temporomandibular disorders are poorly understood, the scientific basis for choice of treatment has not been established. Well-controlled clinical trials comparing various surgical treatments have not been performed. The scientific literature in this field consists mainly of reports based on retrospective studies with small numbers of patients whose outcomes are generally not compared with those of any control group or with those following alternative treatments.

The normal anatomy of the TMJ is relatively well understood. The presence of a biconcave disk interposing between the articular surfaces, which are covered by dense fibrous tissue, allows for smooth function of this synovial joint. Many surgical procedures have been designed to recreate this normal anatomy when internal derangement is associated with TMJ pain or dysfunction, or both. Developments in TMJ imaging techniques, particularly magnetic resonance imaging (MRI), have given us the opportunity to evaluate disk position and anatomy in asymptomatic individuals. This technology has led to the surprising information that internal derangement is common in the asymptomatic population. Surgeons have begun to question the need to reposition a disk, for as many as one third of the general population have anterior disk displacement without signs or symptoms of temporomandibular disorders. The development of arthroscopic techniques for the TMJ led to simple surgical treatments, such as superior joint space lysis and lavage, designed to treat synovial inflammation. These surgical procedures frequently resulted in the return of normal function and a decrease in painful symptoms, but rarely resulted in the repositioning of the disk to a "normal" position between the condyle and the eminence.

Because the arthroscope allows direct inspection of the joint space, changes in synovial tissues can be evaluated. Conditions such as inflammation, adhesions, pseudowalls, and chondromalacia have become commonly described as components of the disease process. In the past, surgeons were worried about the progression from asymptomatic click to symptomatic click to closed-lock to degenerative joint disease. Possible mechanisms are now thought to begin with chronic microtrauma, resulting in inflammation of the synovium combined with poor lubrication of the joint, followed by poor disk mobility, adhesive capsulitis, and the progression of the inflammatory disease process.

In clinical practice, the goals of pain relief and normal functioning of the masticatory apparatus are being achieved by means of techniques such as disk repositioning and arthroscopic surgery. These procedures are designed to restore normal anatomy, treat inflammation, and enhance mobility. Both of these surgical techniques tend to give acceptable clinical results. However, there has been no study comparing these two techniques that might help a given surgeon determine what procedure is indicated in an individual patient. Since temporomandibular disorders are so poorly understood, the goal of treatment should be to provide normal function with minimal pain using the simplest surgical technique available. This retrospective study is designed to compare at a single institution the techniques of disk repositioning by arthrotomy with superior joint space lysis and lavage performed through an arthroscopic technique.

REVIEW OF THE LITERATURE

Disk repositioning surgery has been the most popular technique for open joint procedures. This procedure, also known as plication surgery, has been performed in conjunction with arthroplasty and eminectomy procedures. The therapeutic success of TMJ plication surgery with or without arthroplasty or eminectomy has been reported in the literature.

Mercuri and Campbell[1] performed a postsurgical telephone survey of 21 patients who underwent (1) disk repair, arthroplasty and eminectomy, (2) disk repair and eminectomy, or (3) disk repair and arthroplasty. These authors reported that 91.3% of the patients contacted "felt better," 4.3% "felt the same," and 4.3% "felt somewhat worse." Preoperatively the patients reported an average of 9.3 symptoms each; postoperatively the number of symptoms decreased to 3.2. The results revealed that all procedure combinations except disk repair and arthroplasty gave considerable relief from TMJ pain. Disk repair, arthroplasty and eminectomy provided the most symptomatic relief of the three procedures.

Marciani and Ziegler[2] reported on 51 procedures involving 36 patients who were categorized into one of the following preoperative groups: degenerative joint disease (DJD), hypermobility, hypomobility, and articular disk derangement. The 51 surgical procedures consisted of 22 condylectomies, 11 eminectomies, 12 discoplasties, 4 interpositional gap arthroplasties, and 2 condylar implants. Each patient was sent a questionnaire designed to elicit a perception of the results of surgical treatment. Seventy-seven percent of the respondents reported that their TMJ area discomfort was "much better," and 94% stated they would have surgery again. Fifteen patients had preoperative interincisal openings of less than 35 mm. Of these patients, 11 had a postoperative incisal opening of 35 mm or

more, with a mean increase of 13 mm. The authors concluded that the findings of this study indicate a high percentage of patient satisfaction with the results of TMJ surgery and a general improvement in functional ability.

Dolwick and associates[3] reported a study involving 50 patients (54 joints), with an average follow-up of 24 months. Successful therapeutic results were achieved in 94% of patients following disk repositioning surgery. Tiner and Dolwick[4] reported on 68 patients who had undergone a plication procedure with condylar arthroplasty. Their findings were that 88% of the patients reported excellent or good results, whereas only 12% reported they were worse postoperatively.

Stith[5] reported on 181 patients who had undergone surgical correction of internal derangements and who were followed for 6–42 months. Of 131 patients who had disk repairs, 82% reported marked subjective improvement in symptoms, 10% reported some improvement, 8% reported no improvement, and none reported worsened symptoms. Four percent required further joint surgery.

In 1984 Weinberg reported on 33 patients (40 joints) on whom disk repair and eminectomy were performed.[6] Ninety-six percent of the patients were reported to have improved.

Hall[7] reported on 14 TMJs with anterior disk displacement (ADD) with reduction and 6 TMJs with ADD without reduction that were treated by discoplasty of the superior lamina of the bilaminar zone through the superior joint space. Eminectomies were also performed on each joint. All joints were judged to be markedly improved by both the surgeon and the patients. Sixty-five percent (13) of the joints were pain free, and 37% (7) had mild transient pain with weather changes, prolonged hard chewing, or wide mouth opening. The average postoperative follow-up was 18.1 months.

Kerstens and colleagues[8] performed an eminectomy procedure with or without subsequent discoplasty on 30 patients (36 joints) with internal derangement of the TMJ. The TMJs were clinically evaluated at least 1 year after surgery with respect to opening function and symptoms. The results indicated that 86.8% of the patients "felt better." In 5 patients with a preoperative diagnosis of ADD with reduction, only an eminectomy was performed. This was found to be sufficient to restore normal TMJ function.

A review of articles on TMJ plication with or without arthroplasty or eminectomy for the treatment of internal derangement reveals that the reported success rates range from 77% to 100%. There was, however, no standard for the determination of therapeutic success among the various studies. Even so, disk repositioning surgeries with or without arthroplasty or eminectomy produced excellent therapeutic outcomes and were the preferred treatment for internal disk dysfunction until the advent of TMJ arthroscopic surgery.

In 1975, Ohnishi described the application of arthroscopy to the TMJ for the first time.[9] Later, in the early 1980s, Ohnishi,[10] Kino,[11] and Murakami and Hoshino[12] reported their arthroscopic findings from their studies of cadavers. These authors described anatomic landmarks, reported arthroscopic pathology, and developed useful arthroscopic terminology and regional anatomic nomenclature. Hilsbeck and Laskin[13] and Williams and Laskin[14] conducted arthroscopic surgical experiments on rabbits to determine possible diagnostic applications. In 1980, Ohnishi reported on the clinical application of TMJ arthroscopy as a diagnostic procedure in identifying TMJ disease.[10] Murakami and Ito,[15] Hellsing and coworkers,[16] Burke,[17] Goss and Bosanquet,[18] Tarro,[19] and McCain and colleagues[20] also described the use of TMJ arthroscopy as a diagnostic tool.

Murakami and Hoshino[21] not only discussed the diagnostic application of arthroscopy but also reported on its therapeutic use in the treatment of patients with TMJ closed-lock (ADD without reduction). Murakami described the insertion of a blunt arthroscopic trochar between the fossa and the disk and the movement of the trochar to produce a "sweeping" action resulting in the lysis of fibrous adhesions within the superior joint space. The lysis of adhesions resulted in a mobile disk, and the closed-lock was eliminated.

In 1986, Sanders reported on the therapeutic success of TMJ arthroscopic surgery after performing 40 procedures.[22] He concluded in his article that arthroscopic surgery is a good alternative to arthrotomy. In 1987, Sanders and Buoncristiani again reported on the therapeutic modality of arthroscopic surgery in the treatment of some intracapsular TMJ disorders.[23] They discussed their clinical experience of 137 procedures performed over a 2-year period. Of the 137 arthroscopic procedures, 115 were therapeutic arthroscopies, and 22 were diagnostic only, resulting in immediate arthrotomy. Of the 115 surgical arthroscopies, 94 (82%) were ranked as an excellent result (few or no complaints, an interincisal opening of at least 40 mm, free excursive movements, and few dietary or functional restrictions). A total of 16 (14%) of the 115 surgical arthroscopies were ranked as having good results (minimal or occasional moderate complaints, an interincisal opening of 35 mm or more, and few dietary and functional restrictions). The remaining 5 procedures were ranked as a poor result (moderate to severe complaints, a less than 35 mm interincisal opening, and many functional and dietary restrictions). Overall success was 96% for the 115 therapeutic arthroscopies. Sanders summarized that "therapeutic arthroscopy is an alternative to arthrotomy and can be very effective in eliminating symptoms of preauricular pain and mandibular hypomobility secondary to internal derangement with persistent closed-lock and arthrosis with adhesive capsulitis where nonsurgical therapy has been unsuccessful."

Both Merrill[24] and McCain[25] reported generalized improvement in symptoms in patients with internal derangement following surgical arthroscopy.

Lovasko[26] reported the results of 90 patients with persistent closed-lock managed with surgical arthroscopy over a 2-year period. His results showed a 90% response in the alleviation of the persistent closed-lock condition. A critical analysis of the 90 patients revealed that 49 of them (54%) were classified as having excellent results (no pain, a maximum incisal opening [MIO] of 40 mm or more, and a normal diet). Sixteen patients (18%) were found to have a good result (minimal or occasional pain, a normal diet, and an MIO of 30–35 mm). Twenty-five patients (28%) were regarded as fair or poor (common or continuous pain, a restricted diet, and an MIO of less than 30 mm). Thus, a 72.5% therapeutic success was achieved according to Lovasko's criteria for success.

Dolwick and Nitzan[27] presented a study of 20 patients with a variety of TMJ derangement who underwent lysis and lavage in 28 joints. The patients were evaluated based on a questionnaire. The general success rate was as follows: 16 joints were "better," 9 joints were the "same," and 3 joints were "worse." An overall success rate of 70% resulted. The most impressive results were obtained in patients with displacement without reduction in whom 11 of 12 joints were "better" after surgery. These authors' conclusions were that "patients with painful limitation of opening showed improvement with arthroscopic lavage and lysis of adhesions comparable to results obtained in similar patients with arthrotomy." They continued by stating that "since arthroscopic intervention is less morbid than arthrotomy, arthroscopy is recommended as the initial surgical intervention for patients with painful limited opening."

Israel and Roser[28] performed a study of 25 patients who underwent TMJ arthroscopy with lysis of adhesions and lavage of 28 joints. These patients were evaluated for changes in symptoms and in mandibular opening. The mean follow-up period was 7.5 months. Interviews were conducted in which patients were asked to grade each of their symptoms of pain, joint noise, and jaw opening on a scale of 0–10 (0 indicated that there were no symptoms, and 10 represented the most severe symptoms). Patients evaluated their symptoms preoperatively, 1 month postoperatively, and at monthly intervals thereafter. MIO was also recorded. Preoperatively the mean value for pain was 7.9. One month postoperatively the mean value was 4.5, and in ensuing months was 3.2. A decrease in joint noise from 6.1 preoperatively to 3.4 at 1 month postoperatively, and 3.1 later postoperatively was recorded. There was a decrease in symptoms of restricted jaw opening from 7.1 to 3.2 at later postoperative follow-ups. The results indicated that the patient group had general improvement of the symptoms of pain, joint noise, and mandibular hypomobility following TMJ arthroscopy. Some improvement in symptoms continued beyond the first month into the later postoperative period. There was a 5.9-mm overall improvement in MIO. The authors concluded that arthroscopy appears to be an excellent modality for the management of the symptoms of TMJ pain, joint noise, and limited opening.

Indresano[29] reported the results of an examination of 100 TMJ arthroscopies (64 patients). Eighty joints (50 patients) received a superior compartment sweep and lavage. Three parameters were used to measure success: (1) preoperative and postoperative MIO (a gain of 50% or greater was considered successful); (2) a subjective assessment of pre- and postoperative pain by the patient on a scale of 1–10 (a reduction of pain greater than 70% was considered successful); and (3) the need for additional surgery (any case requiring additional surgery within a 2-year period of the arthroscopic procedure was considered a failure). An overall success rate of 73% was obtained for all surgical arthroscopy procedures. Persistent closed-lock was found to be the most predictably successful condition treated, with a therapeutic success of 83%.

In a multicenter study compiled by Kaminishi and colleagues[30] involving 13 centers and 1344 arthroscopic surgical patients, therapeutic success was based on the reestablishment of good functional movement of the jaws for speaking, eating, and facial expression, and on the reduction of pain so that patients were able to function in a reasonable manner at work and in a home environment. Based on these criteria, therapeutic success was found to range from 70% to 95% with a mean success rate of 87%.

Nitzan and associates[31] evaluated 20 patients who had arthroscopic lysis and lavage with a follow-up of 6 months or greater. The greatest improvement was seen in patients with anterior disk displacement without reduction, and the least improvement was seen patients with ADD with reduction. The authors found their success rates comparable to those for arthrotomy (although a scientific comparison was not presented). They concluded that disk repositioning may be unnecessary to treat TMJ derangement.

Moses and colleagues[32] studied the effect of the arthroscopic release of the TMJ disk in a prospective study using a combination of preoperative tomograms, MRI scans, and arthrograms and postoperative MRI scans. Of the 92 patients evaluated, 60 had bilateral joint disease and 32 had unilateral joint disease. All of the 152 joints studied also had anterior disk displacement preoperatively. Postoperative MRI scans revealed that 92% of the patients had persistent ADD, although 80% of the patients did have marked improvement of disk mobility. Ninety-two percent of the total patient population sampled experienced a significant reduction in pain and the restoration of normal mandibular function. These results reveal that in the vast majority of cases the disk was still anteriorly displaced even though marked improvement of disk mobility did appear to occur.

The therapeutic success of surgical arthroscopy is found to range from 70% to 96%, which is comparable with the results of open joint procedures. However, after an extensive review of the literature, no article has been found to date in which the author made a statistical comparison of the therapeutic success of arthroscopic surgery with arthrotomy and disk repositioning and used this same comparison for the determination of therapeutic success.

METHODS AND MATERIALS

Our study reviewed 63 arthroscopic lysis and lavage procedures of the superior joint space in 47 patients and 79 TMJ arthrotomy and disk repositioning procedures in 59 patients performed at the University of Iowa Hospitals and Clinics. All patients with at least a 6-month follow-up were included in the study. The arthroscopic surgery group was composed of 45 females and 2 males. The mean age for the female patients was 31, with a range of 13–57 years. The males were ages 32 and 43 years. The arthrotomy group consisted of 51 females and 8 males. The average age of the females was 30 years, with a range of 15–50 years. The males had an average age of 28 years, with a range of 20–38 years (Table 8–1). The postoperative follow-up of the arthroscopy patients ranged from 6 months to 2 years, with a mean of 13 months. The longest follow-up for arthrotomy patients was 4.5 years, with a mean of 2.1 years. The median postoperative follow-up for both groups was 14 months.

TABLE 8–1. AGE AND SEX DISTRIBUTION OF ARTHROSCOPY AND ARTHROTOMY PATIENTS

	Males	Females	≤24 Years	25–32 Years	≥33 Years	Total
Arthroscopy	2	45	14	14	19	47
Arthrotomy	8	51	20	20	19	59
Total	10	96	34	34	38	

Preoperative Assessment and Management

Initially, patients presenting with a complaint of TMJ pain or limited opening, or both were examined clinically and radiographically. Once a diagnosis was determined, treatment was initiated. Patients with a diagnosis of internal derangement of the TMJ and who had no previous history of therapy underwent nonsurgical conservative therapy that included nonsteroidal antiinflammatory drugs (NSAIDs), external heat application, physical therapy, splint therapy, or occlusal equilibration, or a combination of these methods. Patients who did not respond to nonsurgical therapy became candidates for surgery. Presurgically, arthrography or MRI was performed as a further adjunct to the diagnosis of the internal derangement. Prior to 1986, the surgical procedure most likely to be performed was arthrotomy with disk repositioning; after 1986, arthroscopic surgical procedures were more common. The decision as to which procedure was eventually performed was made based on the preference of the staff oral surgeon.

Operative Management

TMJ arthroscopic surgery was performed in the operating room with the patient under general anesthesia via nasoendotracheal intubation as an outpatient procedure. Lysis and lavage were performed and followed by injection of betamethasone.

Arthrotomy was performed with the patient under general anesthesia and was usually followed by an overnight admission. A preauricular approach was used to expose the joint. Disk repositioning was accomplished by removing a wedge from the posterior attachment or by folding and oversewing the posterior attachment. In 13 of the 79 procedures, a concomitant eminoplasty was performed using a pneumatic bone file or a manual bone file, or both.

Postoperative Management and Assessment

Postoperative management was individualized for each patient. Patients were asked to initiate self-administered jaw physiotherapy exercises during the first day postoperatively. Those patients with bite appliances were encouraged to wear them if they displayed symptoms. If the patient exhibited nocturnal bruxism, then an occlusal night guard was to be worn. NSAIDs were usually administered for approximately 1 month postoperatively.

Patients were routinely examined at 1 week postoperatively, and thereafter at monthly intervals for 6 months. After this period, annual appointments were arranged if the pain or limited opening resolved. If any complications had arisen from the surgical procedure, patients were reexamined on a more regular basis. Additionally, if their symptoms had recurred, they were instructed to return for further evaluation before the arranged appointment.

Patients were reevaluated at postoperative follow-up visits with respect to preauricular pain, joint noise, interincisal distance, lateral and protrusive movements, and their subjective assessment of postoperative progression.

Several different factors were used in the comparison of arthroscopic and arthrotomic procedures. Factors analyzed included sex; age; the duration of symptoms; the preoperative diagnosis; the type of procedure (unilateral or bilateral); pre- and postoperative pain, noise, and mobility; and prior or subsequent surgical procedures.

Data for the comparative analysis were obtained from the patients' hospital charts. Preoperative data was collected from the initial examinations and the patients' health histories and physical examinations and postoperative data from the operative record and the patients' last follow-up visits.

Assessment of the therapeutic success of an individual procedure was based on the following criteria:

Excellent – An MIO greater than or equal to 35 mm.
– Minimal or no postoperative pain.
– Few or no functional or dietary restrictions.
Good – An MIO of 30–34 mm in breadth.
– Minimal or no postoperative pain.
– Few functional or dietary restrictions.
Poor – An MIO less than 30 mm in breadth.
– Moderate or severe postoperative pain.
– Many dietary or functional restrictions.

A good or excellent result was deemed a therapeutic success.

Based on analysis of the data using a chi-square test, the relative statistical significance for various factors among arthroscopy and arthrotomy and disk repositioning procedures was determined. The results of the comparisons were interpreted as to their clinical relevance to the therapeutic success of the procedures.

In the evaluation of preoperative and postoperative mobility by the two surgical groups (arthroscopy and arthrotomy) for all patients, the parameters for the assessment of MIO were less than 30 mm, 31–37 mm, and greater than 37 mm. These parameters were chosen so that an equal distribution of the number of patients in each parameter could be utilized for statistical comparison of the two surgical groups. In the further evaluation of preoperative and postoperative mobility by the two surgical groups for therapeutic outcome, the parameters followed the criteria for therapeutic success as stated previously, with the exception that the last parameter was divided into two groups (35–39 mm and greater than or equal to 40 mm). The division was performed initially out of a desire to compare the results of the data with those of other studies that used greater than or equal to 40 mm as an excellent result, as opposed to the criterion of greater than or equal to 35 mm as an excellent postoperative result as defined by the American Association of Oral and Maxillofacial Surgery. In this study, the 35–39 mm parameter and the greater than or equal to 40 mm parameter were combined to form the "excellent" category for statistical analysis.

RESULTS

The results of this retrospective study were based on an analysis of the following selected factors used in the comparison of arthroscopy with arthrotomy and disk repositioning.

Sex and Age

A comparison of the 45 female and 2 male arthroscopy patients with the 51 female and 8 male arthrotomy patients with respect to the factors of sex and age revealed no statistically significant difference (Table 8–1). No statistically significant difference was found when arthroscopy and arthrotomy patients were compared with respect to sex and age and therapeutic outcome (Table 8–2).

Duration of Symptoms

In a comparison of arthroscopy and arthrotomy patients with the preoperative duration of symptoms, no statistically significant difference was ascertained. The mean preoperative duration of symptoms for both procedures was approximately 2 years. A comparison of therapeutic outcome with the preoperative duration of symptoms of arthroscopy patients did not reveal any statistical significance (Table 8–3). For these patients, there was an 83% therapeutic success rate for preoperative symptoms with a duration of less than 1 year, a 72% success rate for those lasting 1–4 years, and an 82% success rate for symptoms with a duration greater than 4 years.

A statistically significant difference was demonstrated for arthrotomy patients by comparing the therapeutic outcome with the preoperative duration of symptoms (Table 8–3). Among patients receiving surgery less than 1 year from the onset of symptoms, 88% who underwent arthrotomy and disk repositioning procedures had a therapeutic success. Of these patients, 59% had an excellent result. Eighty-four percent of patients with preoperative symptoms with a duration of 1–4 years had a therapeutic success. However, only 53% of patients with a preoperative duration of symptoms of greater than 4 years had a therapeutic success. Only 12% of the patients with greater than 4 years of preoperative symptoms had an excellent result.

Preoperative Diagnosis

No statistically significant difference was seen between arthroscopy and arthrotomy patients with respect to preoperative diagnosis. Also, no statistical difference was found between a preoperative diagnosis of ADD with reduction and that of ADD without

TABLE 8–2. RESULTS OF ARTHROSCOPY AND ARTHROTOMY PATIENTS BY SEX

	Outcome by Sex for Arthroscopy		
Postsurgical Assessment	*Males*	*Females*	*Total*
Poor	0	10	10 (21.28%)
Good	1	14	15 (31.91%)
Excellent	1	21	22 (46.81%)
Total	2	45	47 (100%)
			p = .718

	Outcome by Sex for Arthrotomy		
Postsurgical Assessment	*Males*	*Females*	*Total*
Poor	3	11	14 (23.73%)
Good	3	16	19 (32.20%)
Excellent	2	24	26 (44.07%)
Total	8	51	59 (100%)
			p = .453

TABLE 8–3. OUTCOME BY PREOPERATIVE DURATION OF SYMPTOMS FOR ARTHROSCOPY AND ARTHROTOMY PATIENTS

	Outcome for Arthroscopy			
	Preoperative Duration of Symptoms			
Postsurgical Assessment	<1 year	1–4 years	>4 years	Total
Poor	7	3	0	10 (21.28%)
Good	8	7	0	15 (31.91%)
Excellent	6	13	3	22 (46.81%)
Total	21 (44.68%)	23 (48.94%)	3 (6.38%)	47 (100%)
Therapeutic Success Rate	83%	72%	82%	p = .099

	Outcome for Arthrotomy			
	Preoperative Duration of Symptoms			
Postsurgical Assessment	<1 Year	1–4 Years	>4 Years	Total
Poor	2	4	8	14 (23.73%)
Good	5	7	7	19 (32.20%)
Excellent	10	14	2	26 (44.07%)
Total	17 (28.81%)	25 (42.37%)	17 (28.81%)	59 (100%)
Therapeutic Success Rate	88%	84%	53%	p = .019

reduction with respect to a particular surgical procedure (Table 8–4). Twenty-nine percent of arthroscopy patients with a diagnosis of ADD with reduction had a therapeutic outcome classified as excellent, 38% had a good outcome, and 33% had a poor outcome. A total therapeutic success of 67% for the treatment of ADD with reduction resulted. However, for patients diagnosed with ADD without reduction, 57% had an excellent therapeutic outcome, 30% had a good result, and 13% had a poor outcome. Overall therapeutic success for ADD without reduction was 87% (Table 8–5).

Forty-nine percent of arthrotomy patients with a preoperative diagnosis of ADD with reduction had a resultant therapeutic outcome classified as excellent, 21% had a good outcome, and 30% had a poor outcome. A 70% therapeutic success rate was seen in patients with ADD with reduction. Thirty-three percent of patients with a preoperative diagnosis of ADD without reduction had a postoperative outcome diagnosed as excellent, 50% had a good outcome; and 17% were diagnosed as poor. The total therapeutic success for ADD without reduction was 83% (Table 8–5).

A 68% therapeutic success rate was found for all patients surveyed with ADD with reduction, and an 85% therapeutic success rate was seen for patients with ADD without reduction. This was a statistically significant difference (p = .03).

Type of Procedure: Unilateral or Bilateral

Thirty-one unilateral and 16 bilateral arthroscopic procedures and 39 unilateral and 20 bilateral arthrotomic and disk repositioning procedures were performed. A comparison of patients undergoing arthroscopy and arthrotomy by unilateral or bilateral procedures revealed that no significant difference existed between the two patient groups. An analysis of therapeutic outcome by type of procedure for arthroscopic surgery patients demonstrated a 90% success rate for unilateral procedures and a 56% therapeutic success rate for bilateral procedures. A chi-square analysis of this comparison was statistically significant (p = .013).

A statistically significant difference (p = .016) was also seen in a comparison of therapeutic outcome and the type of procedure in arthrotomy patients. Eighty-seven percent of unilateral procedures were therapeutically successful, whereas only 55% of bilateral procedures were successful. In an analysis comparing both patient groups by type of procedure, unilateral procedures were found to have a therapeutic success of 89%, whereas only 56% of bilateral procedures were therapeutically successful. Patients who had bilateral procedures were significantly more likely than those having

TABLE 8–4. PREOPERATIVE DIAGNOSIS

Procedure	ADD* With Reduction	ADD* Without Reduction	Both	Total
Arthroscopy	21	23	3	47 (44.34%)
Arthrotomy	33	24	2	59 (55.66%)
Total	54 (50.94%)	47 (44.34%)	5 (4.72%)	p = .461

*ADD = anterior disk displacement.

TABLE 8–5. OUTCOME BY PREOPERATIVE DIAGNOSIS FOR ARTHROSCOPY AND ARTHROTOMY PATIENTS

	Outcome for Arthroscopy			
	Preoperative Diagnosis			
Postsurgical Assessment	ADD* With Reduction	ADD* Without Reduction	Both	Total
Poor	7	3	0	10 (21.28%)
Good	8	7	0	15 (31.91%)
Excellent	6	13	3	22 (46.81%)
Total	21 (44.68%)	23 (48.94%)	3 (6.38%)	47 (100%)
Therapeutic Success Rate	67%	87%		p = .099

	Outcome for Arthrotomy			
	Preoperative Diagnosis			
Postsurgical Assessment	ADD* With Reduction	ADD* Without Reduction	Both	Total
Poor	10	4	0	14 (23.73%)
Good	7	12	0	19 (32.20%)
Excellent	16	8	2	26 (44.07%)
Total	33 (55.93%)	24 (40.68%)	2 (3.39%)	59 (100%)
Therapeutic Success Rate	70%	83%		p = .091

*ADD = Anterior disk displacement.

unilateral procedures to continue to have postoperative pain (p = .001) and limited mobility (p = .007).

In a comparison of all patients with respect to the type of procedure and the duration of symptoms, 17% of the patients who had undergone unilateral procedures had preoperative symptoms for longer than 4 years. However, 44% of the patients who had undergone bilateral procedures had symptoms for longer than 4 years. A chi-square analysis revealed this to be a statistically significant difference (p = .009).

A comparison of the type of procedure and sex; age; preoperative pain, noise, and mobility; additional surgeries; and postoperative pain and noise for all patients revealed no significant difference.

Preoperative Pain

A retrospective analysis of arthroscopy patients showed that 45 patients had preoperative pain and 2 patients had no pain prior to surgery. For arthrotomy patients, 58 patients had preoperative pain and 1 patient was categorized as having minimal pain. No significant difference was found between arthroscopy and arthrotomy patients for preoperative pain. No significant difference was found in a comparison of preoperative pain with therapeutic outcome. Seventy-eight percent of both arthroscopies and arthrotomies in patients with preoperative pain resulted in a therapeutic success.

Preoperative Noise

No statistically significant difference was found in a comparison of preoperative joint noise in the two surgical patient groups. Thirty-three arthroscopy pa-

tients (70%) and 43 arthrotomy patients (73%) had preoperative noise. The postoperative therapeutic success rate for arthroscopy patients was found to be 73% for patients with preoperative noise and 93% for patients with no preoperative noise. Seventy-five percent of arthrotomy patients with preoperative noise experienced a successful outcome, and 81% of patients with no preoperative noise had a therapeutic success. An assessment of all patients revealed that 74% of the patients with preoperative noise and 87% of those with no preoperative noise had a successful therapeutic outcome.

Preoperative Mobility

An evaluation of the two surgical groups showed that no significant difference existed between them with respect to preoperative mobility.

In a comparison of the preoperative mobility of arthroscopy patients with outcome, 73% of patients with a preoperative mobility of less than 30 mm were found to have had a successful outcome. All patients with a preoperative mobility of 30–34 mm had a therapeutic success. There was a 73% success rate for patients with a preoperative opening of 35–39 mm, and a 75% success rate for openings of greater than or equal to 40 mm. No statistically significant differences were seen among the various categories of preoperative mobility as they related to therapeutic success (Table 8–6).

A comparison of therapeutic outcome with preoperative mobility for arthrotomy patients showed an 86% success rate for patients with mobilities of less than 30 mm, a 28% success rate for those with mobilities of 30–34 mm, 87% for those with mobilities of

TABLE 8–6. OUTCOME BY PREOPERATIVE MOBILITY FOR ARTHROSCOPY AND ARTHROTOMY PATIENTS

	Outcome for Arthroscopy				
	Maximum Incisal Opening				
Postsurgical Assessment	*<30 mm*	*30–34 mm*	*35–39 mm*	*≥40 mm*	*Total*
Poor	4	0	3	3	10 (21.28%)
Good	5	3	5	2	15 (31.91%)
Excellent	6	6	3	7	22 (46.81%)
Total	15 (31.91%)	9 (19.15%)	11 (23.40%)	12 (25.53%)	47 (100%)
Therapeutic Success Rate	73%	100%	73%	75%	p = .418

	Outcome for Arthrotomy				
	Maximum Incisal Opening				
Postsurgical Assessment	*<30 mm*	*30–34 mm*	*35–39 mm*	*≥40 mm*	*Total*
Poor	3	5	2	4	14 (23.73%)
Good	10	1	5	3	19 (32.20%)
Excellent	9	1	9	7	26 (44.07%)
Total	22 (37.29%)	7 (11.86%)	16 (27.12%)	14 (23.73%)	59 (100%)
Therapeutic Success Rate	86%	28%	87%	71%	p = .041

35–39 mm, and 71% for patients with preoperative openings greater than or equal to 40 mm. A comparative analysis of preoperative mobility categories showed that the patient group with openings of 30–34 mm (7 patients) was statistically different (p = .041) from the remaining patient preoperative mobility groups. This was, however, a very small sample group, and the relative clinical significance is questionable (Table 8–6). A comparison of outcome based on preoperative mobility for all patients was not found to be of statistical significance.

Postoperative Pain

A comparison of arthroscopy and arthrotomy patients for postoperative pain demonstrated no significant difference between the two groups. Patients were categorized as having continued pain, no pain, or minimal pain. Of the 47 arthroscopy patients, 10 had continued pain, 21 had no pain, and 16 had minimal postoperative pain. Arthrotomy patients displayed similar results, with 13 patients having continued pain, 29 patients having no pain, and 17 having minimal pain.

The therapeutic success rate as it related to postoperative pain was 79% for arthroscopy patients and 78% for arthrotomy patients (Table 8–7). Again, no significant difference between groups was found for therapeutic outcome as it related to postoperative pain. The therapeutic success for all patients based on postoperative pain was 77%.

Postoperative Noise

No significant difference was found between arthroscopy and arthrotomy patients with respect to postop-

TABLE 8–7. OUTCOME BY POSTOPERATIVE PAIN FOR ARTHROSCOPY AND ARTHROTOMY PATIENTS

	Outcome for Arthroscopy Patients			
Postsurgical Assessment	*Pain*	*No Pain*	*Minimal Pain*	*Total*
Poor	10	0	0	10 (21.28%)
Good	0	2	13	15 (31.91%)
Excellent	0	19	3	22 (46.81%)
Total	10 (21.28%)	21 (44.68%)	16 (34.04%)	47 (100%)
Therapeutic Success Rate	0%	100%	100%	
Overall Therapeutic Success Rate	79%			p = .000

	Outcome for Arthrotomy Patients			
Postsurgical Assessment	*Pain*	*No Pain*	*Minimal Pain*	*Total*
Poor	13	0	1	14 (23.73%)
Good	0	3	16	19 (32.20%)
Excellent	0	26	0	26 (44.07%)
Total	13 (22.03%)	29 (49.15%)	17 (28.81%)	59 (100%)
Therapeutic Success Rate	0%	100%	94%	
Overall Therapeutic Success Rate	78%			p = .000

TABLE 8–8. OUTCOME BY POSTOPERATIVE NOISE FOR ARTHROSCOPY AND ARTHROTOMY PATIENTS

Outcome for Arthroscopy Patients			
Postsurgical Assessment	*Noise*	*No Noise*	*Total*
Poor	9	1	10 (21.28%)
Good	9	6	15 (31.91%)
Excellent	9	13	22 (46.81%)
Total	27 (57.45%)	20 (42.55%)	47 (100%)
Therapeutic Success Rate	66%	95%	p = .033

Outcome for Arthrotomy Patients			
Postsurgical Assessment	*Noise*	*No Noise*	*Total*
Poor	8	6	14 (23.73%
Good	5	14	19 (32.20%)
Excellent	10	16	26 (44.07%)
Total	23 (38.98%)	36 (61.02%)	59 (100%)
Therapeutic Success Rate	65%	83%	p = .199

erative noise. However, there was a greater percentage of arthrotomy patients with no noise postoperatively as compared with arthroscopy patients. Sixty-one percent of arthrotomy patients had no postoperative noise, whereas 43% of arthroscopy patients had no postoperative noise.

A significant difference was found with respect to therapeutic outcome when compared with postoperative noise in arthroscopy patients. Patients with postoperative noise had a 66% therapeutic success rate compared with a 95% success rate for patients without postoperative noise (Table 8–8).

The therapeutic outcome of arthrotomy patients as it relates to postoperative noise was not statistically significant, but patients with postoperative noise had a 65% success rate while those without noise had an 83% success rate (Table 8–8).

Assessing therapeutic success based on the postoperative noise results for all patients revealed a 66% success rate for patients with postoperative noise and an 88% success rate for patients with no noise postoperatively.

Postoperative Mobility

The postoperative mobility of arthroscopy and arthrotomy patients was not found to be significantly different. An evaluation of postoperative mobility was performed that measured an increase or decrease in MIO postsurgically. A significant change was deemed to be greater than or equal to 5 mm. Forty-five percent of arthroscopy patients had a postoperative incisal opening showing improvement of greater than or equal to 5 mm as compared with their preoperative baseline mobility. Preoperatively, only 57% of the patients with a postoperative increase in opening were classified as having good or excellent mobility, and just 19% were

categorized as having excellent mobility. Postoperatively, 90% of these patients were classified as having a good or excellent result. Eighty-one percent were found to have an opening characterized as excellent. Forty-two percent had no change in their openings. Ninety-five percent of those patients who experienced no change were postoperatively classified as having good or excellent mobility. Only 13% of the arthroscopy patients had a decrease greater than or equal to 5 mm in their openings. Of those 7 patients who had a decrease in MIO, only 1 was classified as having a poor result (less than or equal to 30 mm). Of the 47 arthroscopy patients, 22 patients were preoperatively categorized with poor or good mobility; they could, therefore, potentially improve their mobility through arthroscopic surgery and attain an excellent classification postoperatively. Thirteen (60%) of the 22 patients that could improve their mobility to a postoperative classification of excellent actually did improve.

Arthrotomy patients were likewise evaluated for postoperative mobility. Forty-nine percent were found to have an increase in MIO. Eighty-six percent of the patients with an increased opening had a good or excellent result. Eighty-three percent were classified with excellent mobility postoperatively. Only 45% of these patients had a preoperative MIO that was classified as good or excellent (35% were excellent and 10% were good). Thirty-one percent had no change in their openings when compared with their preoperative baseline. Ninety-four percent of these patients were already classified as having good or excellent mobility. Twenty percent had a decrease in opening; 4 of these patients (33%) had a poor result. Of the 59 arthrotomy patients, 28 patients could have improved from a classification of poor or good mobility (based on preoperative MIO) to an excellent classification for mobility postoperatively. Fourteen of the 28 patients (50%) had an increase in opening postoperatively of

TABLE 8–9. OUTCOME BY POSTOPERATIVE MOBILITY FOR ARTHROSCOPY AND ARTHROTOMY PATIENTS

	Outcome for Arthroscopy Patients*				
	Maximum Incisal Opening				
Postsurgical Assessment	*<30 mm*	*30–34 mm*	*35–39 mm*	*≥40 mm*	*Total*
Poor	3	1	3	3	10 (21.28%)
Good	3	1	3	8	15 (31.91%)
Excellent	1	1	7	13	22 (46.18%)
Total	7 (14.89%)	3 (6.38%)	13 (27.66%)	24 (51.06%)	
Therapeutic Success Rate	57%	67%	77%	88%	

	Outcome for Arthrotomy Patients†				
	Maximum Incisal Opening				
Postsurgical Assessment	*<30 mm*	*30–34 mm*	*35–39 mm*	*≥40 mm*	*Total*
Poor	4	3	4	3	14 (23.73%)
Good	4	2	10	3	19 (32.20%)
Excellent	1	0	12	13	26 (44.07%)
Total	9 (15.25%)	5 (8.47%)	26 (44.07%)	19 (32.20%)	
Therapeutic Success Rate	56%	40%	85%	84%	p = .02

*Overall therapeutic success rate for arthroscopy patients = 79%.
†Overall therapeutic success rate for arthrotomy patients = 76%.

greater than or equal to 5 mm and were classified as having an excellent result.

Seventy-nine percent of arthroscopy patients who had good or excellent postoperative mobility were considered a therapeutic success (Table 8–9). Seventy-six percent of arthrotomy patients with a good or excellent postoperative mobility had a successful therapeutic outcome (Table 8–9). An assessment of outcome by postoperative mobility for all patients revealed a 72% therapeutic success rate.

Prior or Subsequent Surgical Procedures

Three bilateral arthroscopy patients who underwent an initial arthroscopic surgery with a poor therapeutic result had an excellent therapeutic outcome when they underwent a second arthroscopic procedure.

Nine patients underwent an arthrotomy procedure with a poor postoperative therapeutic outcome. These patients then underwent an arthroscopic surgical procedure. Five of these patients had a poor therapeutic outcome and the other four had a good therapeutic outcome. Thus, 44% of the patients in this group had a successful therapeutic outcome.

Two arthroscopy patients in this study had a poor postoperative outcome and subsequently underwent arthrotomy with disk repositioning. Both patients had a good postoperative result.

Overall Therapeutic Success

A comparison of arthroscopy and arthrotomy patients revealed that 79% of arthroscopy patients and 76% of arthrotomy patients had a postoperative therapeutic success. No significant difference was found between the two groups with respect to therapeutic success.

Complications

Complications were compiled from consecutive populations of 82 arthroscopy patients and 96 arthrotomy patients.

Among the arthroscopic surgery patients were identified five VII nerve deficits, one inferior alveolar nerve paresthesia with a concomitant auriculotemporal nerve deficit, and one anesthesia-related complication. All of these complications resolved over time. Thus, 8% of the patients subsequently developed a postoperative complication.

An assessment of arthrotomy patients revealed five unilateral VII nerve deficits, two bilateral VII nerve deficits, one auriculotemporal paresthesia, two infections, and one upper facial nerve paresis. All of the complications resolved with the exception of the upper facial nerve paresis, which was permanent. Thus, 12% of the patients had postoperative complications.

DISCUSSION

The results of this retrospective study indicate that there was no statistically significant difference between arthroscopy and arthrotomy patients with respect to sex, age, the preoperative duration of symptoms, the preoperative diagnosis, the type of procedure (unilateral or bilateral), or preoperative pain, noise, and mobility. Thus, the two groups were without appreciable differences for preoperative factors, which made it possible to make reasonable comparisons and draw meaningful conclusions as to the therapeutic efficacy of each procedure.

In an analysis of sex and age as preoperative factors used to determine therapeutic success, it was found that neither sex nor age had any bearing on therapeutic outcome for either surgical procedure.

An assessment of the preoperative duration of symptoms for arthroscopy patients revealed that there was an 83% therapeutic success rate for the alleviation of preoperative symptoms lasting less than 1 year, a 72% success rate for those symptoms of 1–4 years in duration, and an 82% therapeutic success for symptoms with a duration greater than 4 years. The success rates for the various time intervals were not significantly different. This would indicate that the therapeutic success of arthroscopic surgery is not dependent on the duration of preoperative symptoms. Therefore, the preoperative duration of symptoms indicating arthroscopy is not a predictive factor for therapeutic success.

A comparison of therapeutic outcome and the preoperative duration of symptoms showed that arthrotomy patients with symptoms lasting less than 1 year achieved an 88% therapeutic success rate and patients with symptoms lasting 1 to 4 years had an 84% success rate. However, arthrotomy patients with symptoms of greater than 4 years in duration achieved only a 53% therapeutic success rate, with only 12% classified as having an excellent result. A statistically significant difference ($p = .019$) was seen in the therapeutic outcome for arthrotomy patients with a preoperative duration of symptoms of greater than 4 years. Therefore, a shorter preoperative duration of symptoms resulted in a more successful outcome for arthrotomy patients. This may be due to the deformation of the disk as a result of its abnormal anterior positioning. The condition of the disk would gradually worsen over time. The restoration of "normal" anatomy by means of arthrotomy and disk repositioning would be difficult owing to permanent disk deformation. The longer the duration of symptoms, the worse the deformation and the more likely the TMJ internal derangement is refractory to treatment. Unlike arthrotomy and disk repositioning surgery, in which the disk is anatomically repositioned, arthroscopic surgery does not result in the repositioning of the disk, but is merely hypothesized to mobilize it. This may account for the therapeutic success of arthroscopic surgery not being affected by a lengthy preoperative duration of symptoms, as a significantly deformed disk may still be able to be mobilized and allow for adaptive joint function.

The therapeutic success of arthroscopy patients with a preoperative diagnosis of ADD with reduction was 67%, and for patients with ADD without reduction it was 87%. For arthrotomy patients, a diagnosis of ADD with reduction resulted in a 70% postoperative success rate as compared with an 83% success rate for patients with ADD without reduction. The increased success rate for the treatment of ADD without reduction in arthroscopy patients may be explained in part by a study by McCain and colleagues,[20] who reported a significantly greater degree of synovial hypervascularity in joints with nonreducing disks as compared with joints with reducing disks.

Hypervascularity is associated with inflammation, and inflammation may result in pain. Therefore, a decrease or the absence of inflammation postoperatively would result in a decrease or the absence of postoperative pain. Arthroscopic surgery serves to increase disk mobility, which would allow for better lubrication of the joint and therefore decrease the potential for joint inflammation. Since surgical arthroscopy does not actually reposition the disk, as revealed in a prospective study performed by Moses and colleagues,[32] (who evaluated pre- and postoperative MRI scans and found that 92% of the patients postoperatively had persistent anterior displaced disks), the treatment of inflammation may be the most significant factor in the treatment of internal derangement, particularly in the case of ADD without reduction.

Another reason for the difference seen in the therapeutic response of patients with ADD with reduction and those with ADD without reduction may be due to the development of fibrotic posterior ligaments resulting from prolonged function. This may result in the creation of a pseudodisk, particularly in the case of a disk without recapture. Less pain would be associated with function on fibrotic tissue, whereas the posterior ligaments, in the case of a reducing disk that is not under constant function, would be less likely to be fibrotic. Function on a nonfibrotic posterior ligament could result in considerable pain, as in the case of ADD with reduction.

An analysis of the therapeutic success of arthroscopy by type of procedure was statistically significant for a 90% success rate for unilateral procedures and a 56% therapeutic success rate for bilateral procedures. Arthrotomy patients had a success rate of 87% for unilateral procedures and 55% for bilateral procedures. These results indicate that unilateral procedures have a greater probability of therapeutic success as compared with bilateral procedures. The reason for this statistically significant difference in success rates ($p = .013$ for arthroscopy and $p = .016$ for arthrotomy) may in part be due to the sheer mathematic significance of dealing with two diseased joints instead of one. All patients having unilateral procedures tended to have symptoms of lesser duration than those having bilateral procedures, so the possibility exists that those having bilateral procedures may have had a more chronic and advanced disease process preoperatively. This advanced disease process may be more difficult to treat. This factor could account for the lower therapeutic success rate observed in patients who underwent arthrotomy procedures with a preoperative duration of symptoms of greater than 4 years. However, there was no difference seen in the therapeutic success of arthroscopy procedures, regardless of the preoperative duration of symptoms. Unilateral procedures also tended to result in significantly greater postoperative mobility than bilateral procedures. The resultant postoperative increase in mobility after unilateral procedures may result in better lubrication and joint function; thus, unilateral procedures have a more successful therapeutic outcome. However, the presence of an intrinsic component in the disease process of patients with bilateral internal derangement, which leads to decreased therapeutic success, cannot be ruled out.

Postoperative pain based on a patient's own subjective assessment and the clinical assessment of the patient's surgeon was found to be similar for both groups, with only 21% of arthroscopy patients and 22% of arthrotomy patients complaining of minimal or significant pain postoperatively.

Arthroscopy patients with postoperative noise had a 66% therapeutic success rate, and those without noise had a 95% success rate. Arthrotomy patients likewise had a higher therapeutic success rate of 83% if they had no postoperative noise, and a 65% success rate if they presented postoperative noise. An absence of postoperative noise was statistically significant for a higher therapeutic success rate for arthroscopic surgery ($p = .033$), but the presence of noise did not preclude a successful outcome. Arthrotomy patients also had a higher success rate for joints without postoperative noise. This finding is associated with the therapeutic success of treating ADD without reduction, which usually manifests as a lack of noise pre- and postoperatively.

An evaluation of postoperative mobility revealed that 60% of arthroscopy patients who were preoperatively classified as having poor or good mobility obtained an excellent mobility after surgery. Fifty percent of the arthrotomy patients with a poor to good mobility improved to achieve an excellent postoperative mobility. These results indicate that disk repositioning is not required to increase postoperative mobility as with the arthroscopic surgery patients. It also indicates that disk mobility may be increased by arthroscopic surgery.

Three patients who underwent arthroscopy with a poor result then underwent a second arthroscopic surgery that resulted in therapeutic success. The success of the second procedure may be due to the inability of the initial arthroscopic procedure to decrease or eliminate the joint inflammation; however, the second procedure successfully decreased inflammation by in-

creasing disk mobility (subsequently increasing lubrication, thereby further decreasing inflammation) or as a result of the injection of additional steroids.

Patients undergoing an arthroscopic surgery secondary to a failed plication procedure did poorly, showing only a 44% therapeutic success rate. The reverse was not true for two patients who initially underwent an arthroscopic surgery and then had a plication procedure. Both had good postoperative results, but the sample size is too small to allow for clinical relevance.

The overall therapeutic success rate of arthroscopic lysis and lavage was 79%, as compared with 76% for arthrotomy and disk repositioning. There was no statistically significant difference between the 2 procedures with respect to their therapeutic outcome.

Reviewing the complications, 8% of the arthroscopy patients and 12% of the arthrotomy patients were found to have postoperative complications. The only permanent deficit occurred after an arthrotomic procedure. Thus, the percentage of postoperative complications was comparable for the 2 groups.

SUMMARY

A retrospective study comparing arthroscopic surgery with arthrotomy and disk repositioning is presented. The therapeutic success rate of arthroscopic surgery was not found to be significantly different from that of arthrotomy and disk repositioning. These results indicate that arthroscopic surgery is an alternative to arthrotomy for certain conditions involving the TMJ. Arthroscopic surgery appears to be effective in eliminating the symptoms of TMJ pain and in restoring mandibular function when nonsurgical therapy has failed, particularly in patients exhibiting ADD without reduction.

Aside from a preoperative diagnosis of ADD with reduction, another factor that may influence the therapeutic success of a procedure is the preoperative duration of symptoms. A shorter preoperative duration of symptoms was found to result in a more successful therapeutic outcome for arthrotomy patients. Early surgical intervention is more likely to result in a successful therapeutic outcome for this procedure.

Yet another factor that contributes to therapeutic success is the type of procedure (unilateral or bilateral). Unilateral procedures resulted in a greater therapeutic success rate than bilateral procedures.

The reason for the success of arthroscopic surgery in the treatment of internal derangement of the TMJ is still only speculative at the present time. Many possible explanations exist. One hypothesis is that, like open joint procedures, arthroscopic surgery functions to reposition the disk and thus restore normal anatomy. This reasoning has been for the most part discounted by studies showing no postoperative change in disk position after arthroscopic surgery. Another explanation is that the therapeutic success is due to the denervation of the joint, which would alleviate joint pain but not necessarily increase mobility. One would expect that after the reinnervation of the joint structures pain would return within a period of several months. This does not appear to be the case, but the possibility exists that during this healing period disk and condylar remodeling may occur, altering the function of the joint to an acceptable environment. The success of surgical arthroscopy may be due to the treatment of joint inflammation by removing the inflammatory substances within the joint, some of which are recognized pain transmitters. Increasing disk mobility would allow for better lubrication of the joint and thereby decrease synovial inflammation. The achievement of disk mobility would also aid in the prevention of adverse loading on the supporting tissues within the TMJ. Further long-term evaluation is still required to better understand the effects of arthroscopic surgery. Other procedures, such as arthrocentesis studies, will help to shed light on the mechanism of arthroscopic surgery's therapeutic effect.

Regardless of its mechanism for therapeutic success, arthroscopic surgery has proved to be of value in the treatment of TMJ internal derangement. As arthroscopic surgery is less morbid than arthrotomy and disk repositioning procedures, but comparable to these procedures in therapeutic outcome, it is recommended for initial surgical intervention in patients with TMJ pain and hypomobility due to internal derangement.

REFERENCES

1. Mercuri, L; Campbell, R; Intra-articular meniscus dysfunction surgery. J Oral Surg (1982), 54:613–621.
2. Marciani, R; Ziegler, R. Temporomandibular joint surgery: A review of fifty-one operations. J Oral Surg (1983), 56:472–476.
3. Dolwick, M; Katzberg, R; Helms, C. Internal derangements of the temporomandibular joint: Fact or fiction? J Prosthet Dent (1983), 49:415.
4. Tiner, BD; Dolwick, MF. Surgical correction of internal derangement of the TMJ: Five-year results. Proceedings of the American Association of Oral and Maxillofacial Surgery Annual Meeting, Las Vegas, Nevada, September 1983.
5. Stith, HE. Surgical treatment of internal derangements of the temporomandibular joint: Review of 198 joints. Lecture presented at the American Association of Oral and Maxillofacial Surgery Annual Meeting, New York, New York, September 1984.
6. Weinberg, S. Eminectomy and meniscoplasty for internal derangements of the temporomandibular joint: Rationale and operative technique. Oral Surg (1984), 57:241.
7. Hall, M. Meniscoplasty of the displaced temporomandibular joint meniscus without violating the inferior joint space. J Oral Maxillofac Surg (1984), 42:788–792.
8. Kerstens, HCJ; Tuinzing, DB; VanDerKwast, WAM. Eminectomy and discoplasty for correction of the displaced temporomandibular joint disc. J Oral Maxillofac Surg (1989), 47:150–152.
9. Ohnishi, M. Arthroscopy of the temporomandibular joint. Kokubyo Gakkai Zasshi (1975), 42:207–213.
10. Ohnishi, M. Clinical application of arthroscopy in the temporo-mandibular joint diseases. Bull Tokyo Med Dent Univ (1980), 27:141–150.
11. Kino, K. Morphological and structural observations of the synovial membranes and their folds relating to the endoscopic findings in the upper cavity of the human temporomandibular joint. Kokubyo Gakkai Zasshi (1980), 47:98–134.
12. Murakami, K; Hoshino, K. Regional anatomical nomenclature and arthroscopic terminology in human temporomandibular joints. Okajimas Folia Anat Jpn (1982), 58:745–760.
13. Hilsbeck, RB; Laskin DM. Arthroscopy of the temporomandibular joint of the rabbit. J Oral Surg (1978), 36:938.
14. Williams, R; Laskin, D. Arthroscopic examination of experimentally induced pathologic conditions of the rabbit temporomandibular joint. J Oral Surg (1980), 38:652–659.
15. Murakami, K; Ito, K. Arthroscopy of the temporomandibular joint. Third report: Clinical experiences. Arthroscopy (1984), 9:49–59.
16. Hellsing, G; Holmlund, A; Nordenram, A; Wredmark, T. Arthroscopy of the temporomandibular joint: Examination of 2 patients with suspected disk derangements. Int J Oral Surg (1984), 13:69–74.
17. Burke, R. Temporomandibular joint diagnosis: Arthroscopy. J Craniomandib Pract (1985), 3:233.
18. Goss, A; Bosanquet, A. Temporomandibular joint arthroscopy. J Oral Maxillofac Surg (1986), 44:614–617.
19. Tarro, A. Arthroscopic diagnosis and surgery of the temporomandibular joint. J Oral Maxillofac Surg (1988), 29:282–289.
20. McCain, J; De la Rua, H; LeBlanc, W. Correlation of clinical, radiographic, and arthroscopic findings in internal derangements of the TMJ. J Oral Maxillofac Surg (1989), 47:913–991.
21. Murakami, K; Hoshino, K. Histological studies on the inner surfaces of the auricular cavities of human temporomandibular joints with special reference to arthroscopic observations. Anat Anz (1985), 160:167.
22. Sanders, B. Arthroscopic surgery of the temporomandibular joint: Treatment of internal derangement with persistent closed lock. Oral Surg Oral Med Oral Pathol (1986), 62:361–372.
23. Sanders, B; Buoncristiani, R. Diagnostic and surgical arthroscopy of the temporomandibular joint: Clinical experience with 137 procedures over a two-year period. J Craniomandib Dis Fac Oral Pain (1987), 1:202–213.
24. Merrill, R. Operative arthroscopy experiences. Presented at the First Annual International Symposium on Arthroscopy of the Temporomandibular Joint, New York, New York, July 1986.
25. McCain, JP. Operative arthroscopy. Lecture presented at the First Annual International Symposium on Arthroscopy of the Human Temporomandibular Joint, New York, New York, July 1986.
26. Lovasko, J. Results in the arthroscopic surgical management of 90 patients with persistent closed lock. Lecture presented at the Third Annual International Symposium on Arthroscopy of the Human Temporomandibular Joint, New York, New York, December 1988.
27. Dolwick, MF; Nitzan, DW. TMJ arthroscopic lavage and lysis of adhesions: Preliminary report. Lecture presented at the Third Annual International Symposium on Arthroscopy of the Human Temporomandibular Joint, New York, New York, December 1988.
28. Israel, H; Roser, S. Patient response to temporomandibular joint arthroscopy: Preliminary findings in twenty-four patients. J Oral Maxillofac Surg (1989), 47:570–573.
29. Indresano, A. Arthroscopic surgery of the temporomandibular joint: Report of sixty-four patients with long-term follow-up. J Oral Maxillofac Surg (1989), 47:439–441.
30. Kaminishi, R; Davis, C; Moses, J. A multicenter study and the evaluation of the efficacy of arthroscopic surgical procedures of the temporomandibular joint. Lecture presented at the Fifth Annual International Symposium on Arthroscopy of the Temporomandibular Joint. New York, New York, December 1990.
31. Nitzan, D; Dolwick, F; Heft, M. Arthroscopic lavage and lysis of the temporomandibular joint: A change in perspective. J Oral Maxillofac Surg (1990), 48:798–801.
32. Moses, J; Satoris, D; Glass, R; et al. The effect of arthroscopic surgical lysis and lavage of the superior joint space on TMJ disc position and mobility. J Oral Maxillofac Surg (1989), 47:674–678.

Nine

Temporomandibular Joint Arthroscopic Surgery
The Endaural Approach, Lateral Eminence Release, Capsular Stretch, and Articular Eminoplasty—Rationale and Technique

JEFFREY J. MOSES, D.D.S.
DANIEL C. TOPPER, D.D.S.

Since Ohnishi's[1] 1975 development of a puncture technique for the penetration of the temporomandibular joint (TMJ) using a small arthroscope, major advances have been made in the arthroscopic diagnosis and treatment of TMJ pathology. Inspection of the superior joint compartment has traditionally been accomplished via the superior anterolateral or the superior posterolateral portals. However, certain limitations of these traditional approaches have become evident, especially when the lateral trough and the anterolateral joint space are visualized or when access to the medial and the lateral paradiscal troughs is required for instrumentation. Clear visualization of these areas is impeded when currently available 15-degree angled scopes are used and when lateral approaches are employed. On the contrary, endaural entry makes possible clear visualization and the uncluttered use of instrumentation in the surgery of the medial and especially the lateral TMJ spaces.

THE ENDAURAL APPROACH

Ohnishi described the endaural puncture originally in 1982 and again in 1986.[2,3] Modifications and refine-ments of this technique have also been reported by this author.[4,5] The technique of endaural access is relatively simple, but it does require attention to basic technical points if complications are to be prevented. First, the joint should be fully distended to facilitate trocar puncture and to minimize the risk of iatrogenic intracapsular damage. Second, the skin should only be punctured with a sharp trocar. Third, all intraarticular procedures should be performed with care to prevent articular surface damage. Finally, the joint space should be kept expanded by a slow-infusion irrigating system.

A 30-degree angled arthroscope is recommended when performing this technique. An instrument of this size provides the surgeon increased panoramic visualization of the joint. The off-axis viewing angulation changes as the scope is rolled. This allows for a more comprehensive examination of the joint in areas difficult to examine with the conventional 15-degree arthroscope. In the visualization of the lateral capsule and attachment areas it is important to use an arthroscope that has its visual access oriented toward the light cord. This makes it possible to prevent the light cord from becoming pressed against the patient's temporal area. As this feature constitutes a deviation from the usual manufacturer's product design, it must be specifically requested by the surgeon when the arthroscope is ordered.

Technique

The operative site, including the external auditory meatus (EAM), is prepared using an aseptic technique. A packing of the ear is accomplished after preparation. The superior joint space is initially penetrated from the standard superior posterolateral approach. The arthroscope is angled and rotated, so that the light shines through the anterior wall of the external acoustic meatus. This spot is usually located 1.0–1.5 cm medial to the lateral edge of the tragus in the EAM (Fig. 9–1).

With the mandible distracted downward and forward, the anterior wall of the external auditory canal is perforated with the sharp trocar and the 30-degree arthroscopic cannula. The cannula and trocar are angled anterosuperiorly and slightly medially, perpendicular to the posterior slope of the articular eminence and *above* the level of the superior posterolaterally placed arthroscope. This ensures the puncture of the superior compartment (Fig. 9–2).

The depth of penetration of the superior joint compartment should be no greater than 1.5 cm. Confirmation of penetration is made by direct visualization of the trocar and of the outflow of irrigating fluid from the endaural cannula when the trocar is removed. The arthroscope is inserted into the endaural cannula, and the inflow tubing is connected. The superior posterolateral cannula is then sealed with a small rubber cap to prevent excessive outflow. The cannula can be utilized as a working portal while visualization is accomplished via the endaural scope.

The medial, lateral, and superior aspects of the joint are examined by rotating the arthroscope and holding the camera steady. This approach is especially helpful when visualizing the anterolateral synovial space, and it allows the superior posterolaterally and superior anterolaterally placed cannulas to be used for instrumentation.

At the completion of the procedure the cannulas are removed. The lateral punctures may be dressed with small, round adhesive bandages. The endaural puncture site is left undressed (the elastic cartilage closes the entry site). A routine otoscopic examination is usually performed postoperatively after removal of the ear pack in order to visualize the EAM and tympanic membrane and to confirm that the procedure caused no damage. Finally, the patient is administered polymyxin B sulfate-neomycin sulfate-hydrocortisone (CORTISPORIN) otic suspension for three days postoperatively to prevent otitis externa.

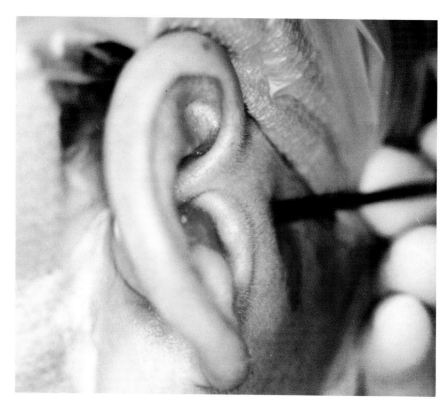

FIGURE 9–1. Endaural transmeatal illumination via the superior posterolateral (SPL) arthroscope portal.

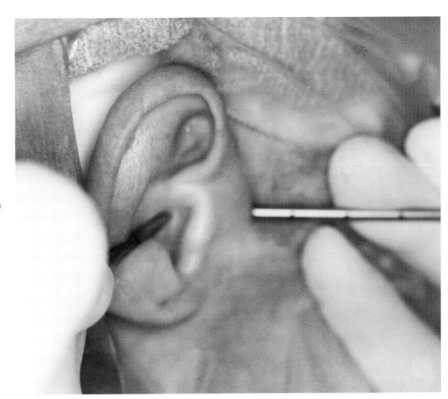

FIGURE 9–2. Endaural puncture location point and angle/depth.

THE LATERAL EMINENCE RELEASE

Rationale

The pathophysiology of progressive disk displacement and lateral impingement phenomenon has been previously reported.[4] We have learned that the majority of pathologic adhesions and sources of restricted disk motion are found within the lateral one third of the joint. The soft tissues of the capsule become fibrotic and constricted due to inactivity or inflammation, thereby restricting mandibular movements. Inflamed synovial proliferation and projection as well as adhesions binding the disk to the eminence and capsule—factors leading to restricted mobility—are frequently observed from the endaural view looking forward along the superior lateral compartment trough. In our clinical studies we found that lateral eminence release and capsular stretch procedures combined with routine arthroscopic lysis of adhesions and lavage relieved pain and reduced the restriction of mandibular mobility in more than 92% of the patients diagnosed with immobile articular disks.[6]

Objective

The objectives of lateral eminence release are (1) to release lateral impingement and to arrest adhesive capsulitis, (2) to stretch the fibrosed or constricted capsule and the TMJ ligament, (3) to mobilize the condyle-disk unit for greater translatory glide of the superior joint compartment, and (4) to give physical therapists a head start in their management of restricted range of motion.

Technique of Lateral Eminence Release and Capsular Stretch

The technique can be performed under direct visualization via the endaural portal. Alternatively, the release can be accomplished indirectly from within the superior joint compartment by utilizing either the superior anterolateral or the posterolateral portal to perform the lysis of adhesions, the sweep of the lateral tubercle and eminence, and the lateral stretch of the capsule (Fig. 9–3).

A hardened, blunt trocar is inserted into a cannula placed in the superior joint compartment via the superior posterolateral portal. The glenoid fossa is gently palpated, and the trocar is advanced anterior to the posterior slope of the articular eminence. The trocar is then pulled laterally over the lateral articular eminence, thereby stretching the capsule and sweeping the lateral capsular adhesions (Fig. 9–4).

As the lateral margin of the lateral eminence is palpated, the trocar is directed superiorly, releasing

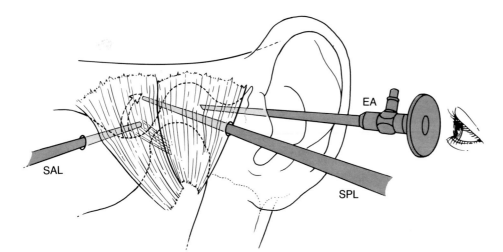

FIGURE 9–3. Visualization via the endaural (EA) portal with lateral eminence release (LER) from the superior posterolateral (SPL) or superior anterolateral (SAL) portal. (From Thomas, M; Bronstein, S. Arthroscopy of the Temporomandibular Joint. Philadelphia: W.B. Saunders Co. (1992), 196.)

the superior lateral capsular attachments. The surgeon's free hand is placed on the outer skin surface for bimanual palpation of the extent of lateral capsular stretch and lateral capsular release from the articular tubercle.

Débridement may follow via either the superior anterolateral portal or the superior posterolateral portal. Finally, the arthroscope is reintroduced into the superior joint compartment. Disk mobility is confirmed on condylar translation.

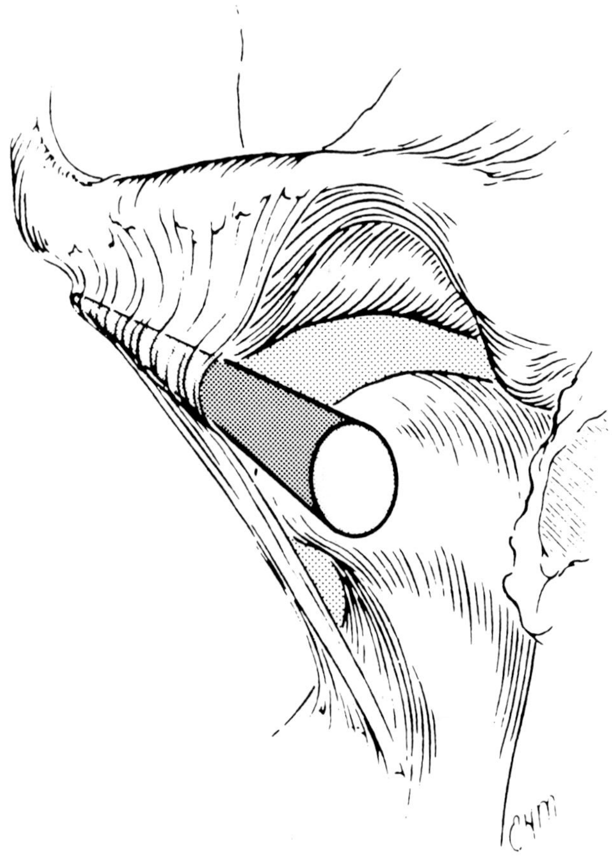

ARTICULAR EMINOPLASTY

Rationale

The impingement syndrome of the shoulder is well known to orthopedic surgeons. Neer[7] demonstrated an impingement between the anterior edge of the acromion and the coracoacromial ligament on the forward elevation of the shoulder. His findings are well supported by his studies of cadavers, which demonstrate bony changes consisting of roughness, erosion, and osteophyte formation on the anteroinferior surface of the acromion in older subjects. Internal rotation in the forward flexed position tends to drive the greater tuberosity further under the coracoacromial arch, so that the impingement area comes directly under the coracoacromial ligament. When the arm is forcibly flexed forward, pain occurs. Treatment directed toward reducing inflammation includes the use of ice, ultrasound, and antiinflammatory agents. Physical therapy programs aimed at increasing flexibility and strength are also pursued. Surgical decompression, accomplished by resecting the corocoacromial ligament, or a more definitive anterior acromioplasty, may be indicated in severe cases.[8]

A similar problem may occur in the TMJ. In cases of long-standing lateral capsular prolapse, hypertrophic articular tubercles are often seen in conjunction with areas of lateral condylar resorption when the condyles are viewed in a protruded position on coronal tomograms. If the joint space diminishes with degenerative changes, the condyle articulates more heavily at the lateral area during protrusive and opening movements, with painful impingement resulting on the lateral one third of the disk (Fig. 9–5). This can be seen particu-

FIGURE 9–4. Posteroanterior view of the lateral capsular stretch (LCS) from a superior posterolateral portal, reversing the effect of capsular fibrosis on mobility.

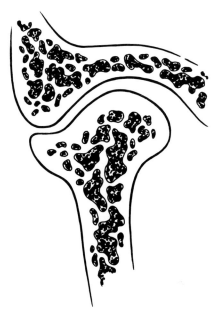

FIGURE 9–5. Coronal view of a degenerated condyle in the protruded jaw position articulating with the hypertrophied lateral tubercle of the eminence.

larly well from the endaural view along the lateral trough (Figs. 9–6, 9–7, and 9–8). The impingement is confirmed by our observation that disk perforation is most frequently observed at the lateroposterior bilaminar zone–disk junction (Fig. 9–9).

The technique of lateral eminence release is employed to release adhesions and to stretch the lateral capsule. In addition, eminoplasty is required to reduce the hypertrophic articular tubercle, thereby creating more joint space and limiting the recurrence of the impingement syndrome.

Technique

First, capsular stretch and lateral eminence release are performed as previously described. The arthroscope is then inserted into the superior joint compartment via the endaural approach, utilizing a reverse 30-degree cannula. Fibrous tissue tags are visualized over the lateral eminence where release was accomplished.

The arthroscopic light is directed laterally, providing a target for the superior anterolateral puncture. The anterior puncture distance may be determined by measuring the calibration marks on the endaural cannula and by aligning the sharp superior anterolateral trocar in a parallel manner. This will ensure a puncture anterior to the scope, facilitating triangulation (Figs. 9–10 and 9–11).

By turning the trocar and the cannula 90 degrees to the skin surface and by aiming several millimeters ahead of the illumination (Figs. 9–12 and 9–13), the superior anterolateral puncture is made. Entry into the superior joint compartment is confirmed both by means of the scope and by the presence of irrigation return

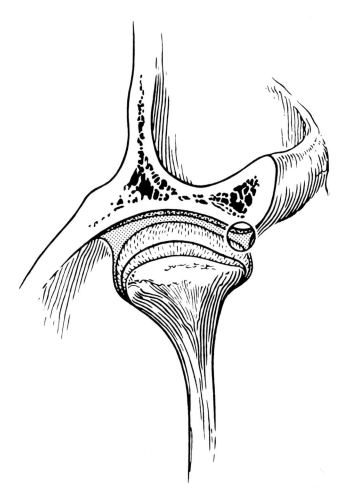

FIGURE 9–6. Coronal view of the temporomandibular joint with a circle highlighting the lateral trough and the area where impingement is most likely to occur.

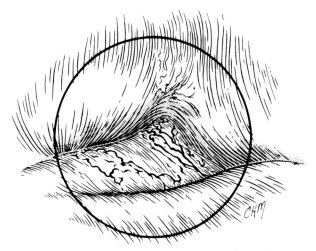

FIGURE 9–7. Illustration of the hypertrophied lateral tubercle impinging on the articular disk and attachment capsule as viewed from the endaural portal.

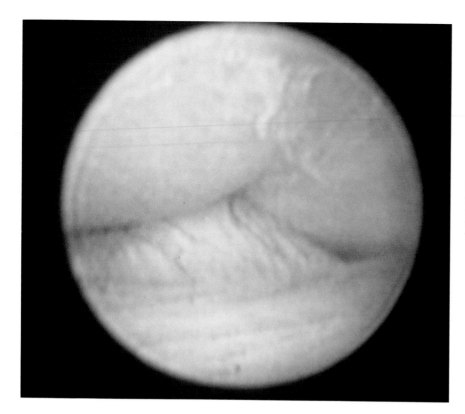

FIGURE 9–8. Arthroscopically assisted photograph of a hypertrophied lateral tubercle with impingement syndrome. Note: Synovial hypervascularity (creeping synovitis) of the lateral attachment to the disk is present.

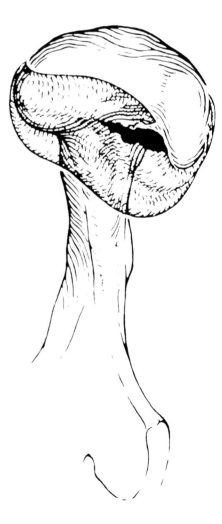

FIGURE 9–9. Illustration of the disk–condyle complex is viewed anterosuperiorly with perforation present in the lateral third of the anteriorly displaced disk at its bilaminar attachment.

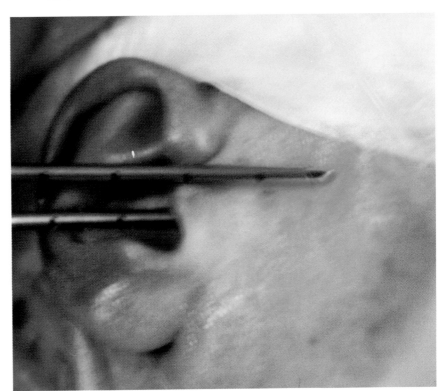

FIGURE 9–10. Transcutaneous illumination along the lateral trough yielding guidance for cannula measurement and placement.

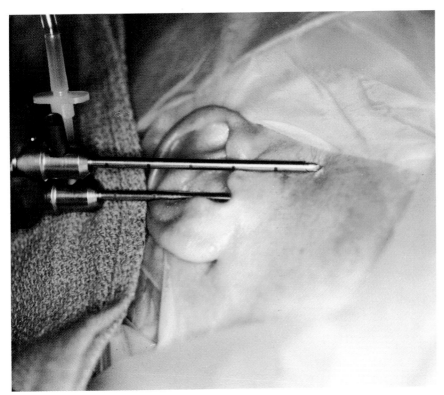

FIGURE 9–11. Parallel cannula length measurement technique allowing precise guidance of puncture distance anteriorly.

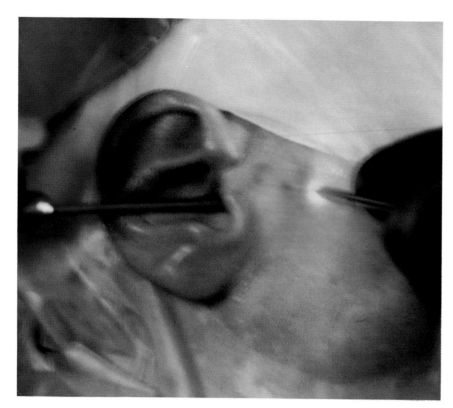

FIGURE 9–12. Endaurally placed arthroscope giving exact transcutaneous illumination for the superior anterolateral (SAL) trocar/cannula puncture.

FIGURE 9–13. Demonstrated finger-protected superior anterolateral (SAL) trocar/cannula positioned perpendicularly to the skin.

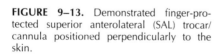
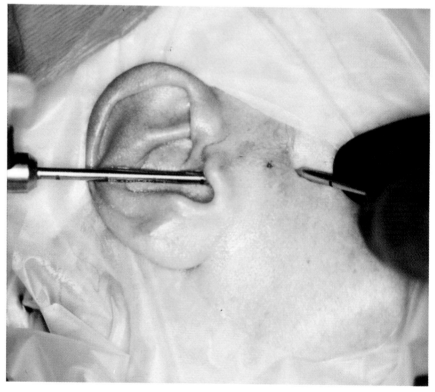

on removal of the trocar from the cannula. The superior anterolateral cannula may now be removed. The shaver sheath of a power abrader is inserted through the previously formed cannula tract into the superior joint compartment.

Utilizing the endaural portal for visualization and the superior anterolateral portal for instrumentation, the fibrocartilaginous remnants of the articular eminence are carefully removed. For maximum cutting efficiency, a setting of 25–50% power is recommended. This speed produces a low level of suction and helps to keep the débrider blades clean. The shaver may be rotated to débride the synovium and the disk. Débridement of the lateral eminence is continued until bone is reached.

Power-assisted eminoplasty requires maximum distraction of the joint. This is accomplished by utilizing an arthroscopic joint spreader/stabilizer (Fig. 9–14). The zygomatic arch over the articular tubercle is palpated, and a needle, directed perpendicular to the skin, is inserted to the bone (Fig. 9–15). The needle depth is marked and measured. Five millimeters is added to the depth measurement to ensure bone penetration by the stabilizing pin (Fig. 9–16). This measurement is then transferred to the threaded K-wire (Kirschner wire), and a rotary bur is used to mark the K-wire at that depth (Fig. 9–17). Utilizing the same

needle puncture tract, a 0.062 threaded K-wire is drilled into the zygomatic arch at the premeasured depth marked on the surface of the pin. The measurement procedure is repeated at the condylar neck. An additional 0.062 threaded K-wire is drilled at this location after first pinching and gathering the skin between the sites together. This produces the flexibility needed for spreading following pin placement. The arthroscopic joint spreader/stabilizer is then placed over the K-wires and the joint is distracted (Fig. 9–18).

Visualization and operative access may now be accomplished by any combination of the superior anterolateral, superior posterolateral, and endaural approaches (Figs. 9–19 and 9–20). It is interesting to note that the superior joint compartment does not increase in size until irrigation fluid is introduced. The hydraulic action of the fluid helps push the disk inferiorly against the condyle.

The abrader bur and cannula are introduced into the previously dilated superior anterolateral portal (Fig. 9–21). Under direct observation the hypertrophic articular tubercle is reduced by gently moving the abrader bur in sweeping strokes. After an appropriate level of reduction is achieved, the cannula and abrader are removed. A hand or power file or rasp is then utilized to smooth the abraded area (Fig. 9–22).

The joint spreader is now removed along with the

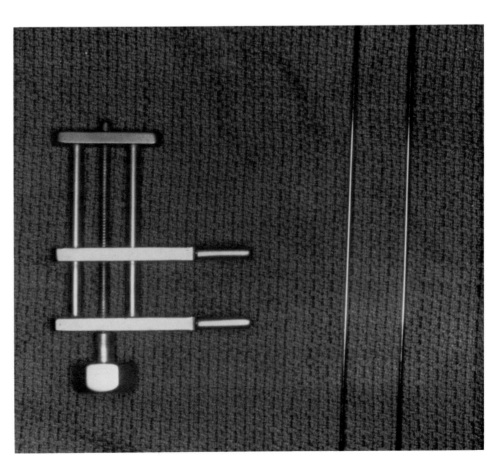

FIGURE 9–14. Arthroscopic joint spreader/stabilizer and 0.062 pins.

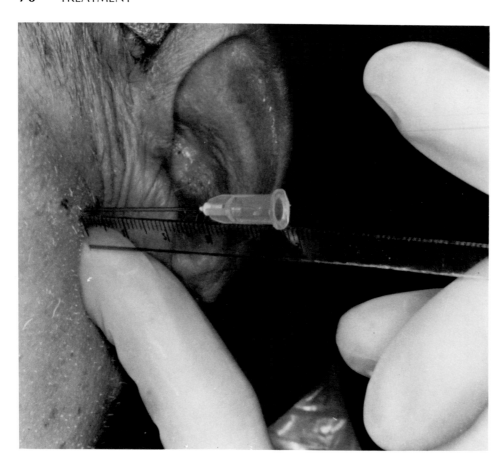

FIGURE 9–15. Needle-guided depth measurements of zygomatic arch and condyle.

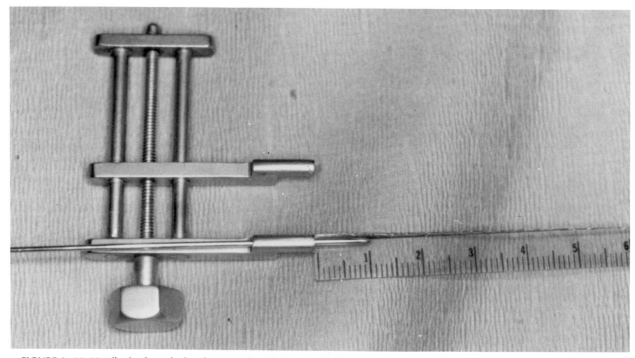

FIGURE 9–16. Needle depth marked and measured, with 5 mm added to the depth to ensure bone penetration of the stabilizing pin.

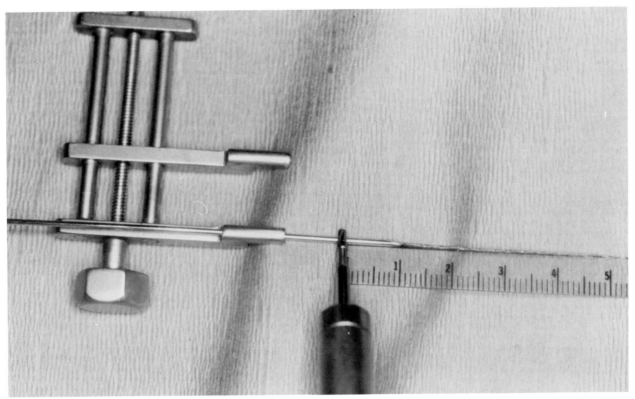

FIGURE 9–17. Rotary bur used to transfer the mark to the pin for reference.

FIGURE 9–18. Arthroscopic joint spreader/stabilizer with superior anterolateral (SAL) abrader and end-aural (EA) arthroscope in place.

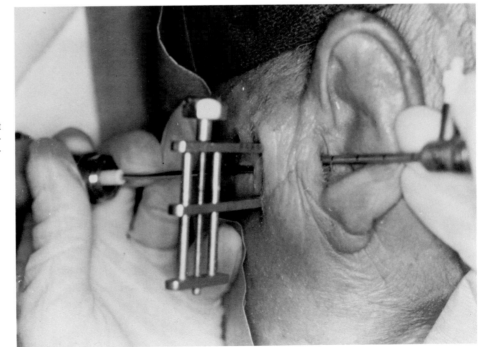

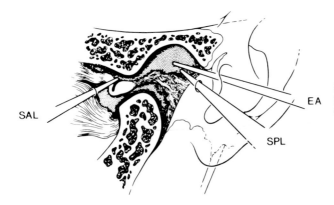

FIGURE 9–19. Various locations of the superior joint compartment access portals: superior anterolateral (SAL), superior posterolateral (SPL), and endaural (EA).

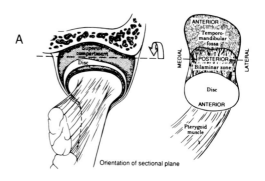

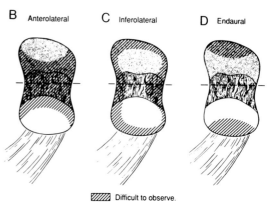

FIGURE 9–20. Areas of the visual fields with each of the superior joint compartment portals.

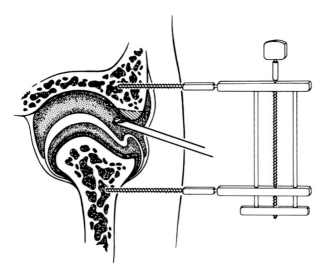

FIGURE 9–21. Coronal view of temporomandibular joint eminoplasty with the joint spreader/stabilizer in place.

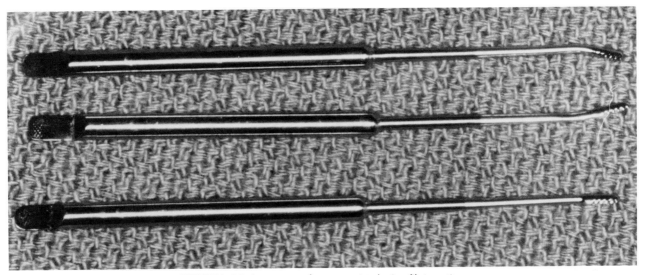

FIGURE 9–22. Assortment of power-assisted microfile/rasp tips.

K-wires. A superior posterolateral cannula is left in the superior joint compartment, and lavage of the joint is performed with an iced, heparinized solution. Two thousand IU of heparin are added to one liter of solution to aid in the prevention of clots that could block the outflow portal. Simultaneously, the assistant "pumps" the joint by manual movement of the mandible.

The arthroscope is reintroduced into the superior posterolateral cannula, and the mobility of the disk on condylar translation is confirmed. Visualization of the lateral eminence area by the endaural approach confirms the elimination of lateral impingement by the tubercle. The cannulas are removed, and the lateral puncture sites are dressed with round adhesive bandages. Finally, the external auditory canal and tympanic membrane are inspected for damage.

SUMMARY

Pathologic adhesions cause a change in disk/condyle dynamics and lead to pain and dysfunction. The majority of motion-restricting pathologic adhesions within the TMJ appear to occur in the lateral aspect of the joint. Capsular tissues become fibrotic and constricted secondary to mediolateral torsional displacement of the disk at the head of the condyle and postinflammatory healing changes. Perforations of the junction of the posterolateral disk and the bilaminar zone are consistent with this hypothesis. Arthroscopy via the inferolateral, superior posterolateral, or superior an-

terolateral approaches may not allow visualization of the lateral trough of the joint. Utilizing the endaural approach, a nearly direct posterior access is possible, allowing visualization of the lateral capsule. Relief of the restraints on disk/condyle dynamics is accomplished via the capsular stretch technique and lateral eminence release technique. Finally, hypertrophic articular eminences and tubercles occasionally require reduction to prevent discal or capsular impingement during translatory or excursive mandibular movement. The technique of articular eminoplasty is employed to achieve this goal.

REFERENCES

1. Ohnishi, M. Arthroscopy of the temporomandibular joint. Kokubyo Gakkai Zasshi (1975), 42:207–213.
2. Ohnishi, M. Clinical studies on the intra-articular puncture of the temporomandibular joints and its application. Kokubyo Gakkai Zasshi (1982), 31:487–512.
3. Ohnishi, M. Arthroscopic pathological findings and surgical procedures. Proceedings of the Symposium on TMJ Arthroscopy and Arthroscopic Surgery, Oral and Maxillofacial Surgery Foundation, Long Beach, California, 1986.
4. Moses, J. Lateral impingement syndrome and endaural surgical technique. Oral Maxillofac Surg Clin N Am (1989), 1:175–183.
5. Moses, J; Poker, I. Temporomandibular joint arthroscopy: The endaural approach. Int J Oral Maxillofac Surg (1989), 18:347–351.
6. Moses, J; Poker, I. TMJ arthroscopic surgery: An analysis of 237 patients. J Oral Maxillofac Surg (1989), 47:790–794.
7. Neer, CS. Anterior acromioplasty for the chronic impingement syndrome in the shoulder: A preliminary study. J Bone Joint Surg (1972), 54:41–50.
8. Hawkins, RM; Kennedy, JC. Impingement syndrome in athletes. Am J Sports Med (1980), 8:151–158.

Ten

Arthroscopic Temporomandibular Joint Lysis, Lavage, and Manipulation and Chemical Sclerotherapy for Painful Hypermobility and Recurrent Mandibular Dislocation

R.G. MERRILL, D.D.S., M.Sc.D.

This chapter presents a conservative surgical method for the treatment of patients with symptomatic hypermobility or recurrent mandibular dislocation. Patients with one of these disorders who were included in this study had disk derangements of malposition and deformity. The method combines the old technique of injecting a sclerosing agent with the newer technology of temporomandibular joint (TMJ) arthroscopic surgery. This procedure was initially performed in those with recurrent mandibular dislocation, and subsequently in those with painful hypermobility. The treatment objectives were to improve mandibular function, to reduce joint laxity, and to alleviate pain and other associated symptoms.

Hypermobility of the mandible in association with internal derangement of the disk is quite common. However, the incidence of recurrent mandibular dislocation is only approximately 3%. The three types of chronic mandibular anterior dislocation are long-standing, recurrent, and habitual. This study includes patients with anterior recurrent dislocation. Condylar

subluxation is an incomplete dislocation in which articular surfaces maintain partial contact. The patient with condylar subluxation is able to return the condyle to the glenoid fossa voluntarily by self-manipulation. An incomplete transient dislocation (subluxation) can occur when the condyle becomes temporarily blocked in its path of closure either in front of the disk or by a deformation of the disk. Advanced degenerative disease combined with the presence of rough articular surfaces can be associated with condylar subluxation and luxation. Joints may be predisposed to subluxations, dislocations, and internal derangements involving the disk by virtue of their hypermobility.

Hypermobility without symptoms can be considered normal for a large segment of the population. It is characterized by a strong forward movement of the condyle when the mouth is fully opened with absence of symptoms or strain during either opening or closing movements. This is the only joint in the body that gives the appearance of a dislocation in lateral radiographic images. The condyle depicted in the radiograph

75

of the open mouth is situated anterior to the articular eminence. The mouth can be closed without locking, clicking, or other signs and symptoms. Hypermobility becomes clinically significant when signs and symptoms are present. It is rare to identify patients with either painful hypermobility or recurrent dislocation who do not have an associated disk derangement. Other hypermobile joints that become symptomatic have been referred to as having a *hypermobility syndrome*.

REVIEW OF THE LITERATURE

Schultz[1] was the originator of sclerotherapy for hypermobility and recurrent dislocation of the TMJ. He reported on his animal studies and clinical applications in 1937. Sodium psylliate was injected into the TMJ cavities of 12 dogs every 2 weeks for 3 months. There were 8–10 injections in each joint. At autopsy, the cartilage surfaces and the synovial membrane were smooth and glistening. All joints were judged to be in excellent functional and anatomic condition. The joint capsules measured 5–7 mm more in thickness than those of the control specimens. There were no gross changes in the ligaments other than thickening. Subacute reaction with infiltration of leukocytes followed 30 minutes after the injection. Two hours later lymphocytic infiltration was begun. Fibrosis started after 4–6 days. A 5% loss in the size of the original opening was noted.

Schultz made other pertinent observations relating to the injection of sodium psylliate at other anatomic sites in the animals. Subcutaneous injections up to 20 ml resulted in large areas of firm fibrosis without sloughing after 3 weeks. The injection of 1–2 ml into abdominal scars caused a small area of necrosis. Injections into the mental and the infraorbital nerves and into other motor nerves produced no effect. Injection into the blood stream and the heart also produced no recognizable effects. No infections were noted. In his clinical applications Schultz injected 0.5 ml of sodium psylliate into the superior joint cavity with the condyle in the wide-open position. The goal of the procedure was to thicken and shorten the joint capsule using the fibrosing agent. Injections were repeated weekly until sufficient fibrosis was achieved. (This required 3–4 injections.) Prior to 1937, 30 joints were treated with complete satisfaction and no complications.

In 1947 Schultz[2] reported on 10 years of experience in treating hypermobility of the TMJ using 5% sodium psylliate sclerosing solutions combined with a local anesthetic. He directed attention to the simplicity and safety of the method for the treatment of joints with lax ligaments. Later, in 1943, Schultz and Shriner[3] reported on their success in using the sclerosant in 200 patients. In 1941 Moose[4] injected 0.5 ml of a 5%

sodium psylliate solution into the mandibular joint cavities of three rhesus monkeys weekly for 1 year, confirming the animal research performed by Schultz.[1] There were no deleterious effects. Moose was an advocate of using sodium psylliate in humans with hypermobility. He advised continued postinjection mandibular function, restrained but not fixed opening, and the strengthening of the tissues responsible for limiting condylar movement.

In 1950, McKelvy[5] reported on his use of a 0.5-ml emulsion of a 5% sodium psylliate solution injected into the superior joint cavity of 100 patients. He found that 75% were cured, 9% were improved, 5% had questionable improvement, and 11% failed. The average treatment period was 1 month, with most patients requiring three injections 1–2 weeks apart. Postoperatively the patients were advised to avoid wide opening. Intermaxillary fixation was not used.

Later, Thoma[6] injected 1 ml of a 5% sodium psylliate solution into the superior joint compartment of patients with hypermobility, terminal clicking, recurring subluxation, and a slack capsule but without trismus. Intermaxillary fixation was not used, but patients were advised to avoid wide mouth opening as Schultz,[2] Moose,[4] and McKelvy[5] had advocated.

In 1975 Archer[7] performed a survey of the use of sclerosing solutions in the treatment of TMJ disorders. This was prompted by a controversial panel discussion on treatment of subluxation and dislocation at the 1975 annual meeting of the Great Lakes Society of Oral Surgeons. One hundred twenty-two of the surgeons replied to the survey, 60 of whom reported using sclerosing injections for the treatment of hypermobility. There was a cumulative 1055 years of experience in the use of this procedure by the 60 surgeons. The complications of persistent pain and excessive limitation of mandibular motion as well as radiographic evidence of articular degeneration were reported by 6 of the surgeons, but no specifics as to the number of complications were provided. There were 37 predominantly favorable anecdotal comments from the surgeons, most of whom commented on the absence of any deleterious effects caused by the sclerosing injection. For example, Dr. Schultz responded, "I am the originator of this type of treatment. I have injected thousands of cases with only good results. I have retired and would offer to debate any and all men who make statements against injection therapy."

Ohnishi and colleagues,[8,9] the originators of arthroscopy of the TMJ, have reported on the use of the arthroscopic technique for either electrocautery or Nd:YAG (neodymium-yttrium-aluminum-garnet) laser scarification of the oblique protuberance area in patients with hypermobility and recurrent mandibular dislocation. The oblique protuberance is a prominent fold running from the disk attachment area of the medial pole of the condyle to the posteromedial wall of the glenoid fossa and is visible when the condyle is translated forward in the posterior superior synovial pouch. The arthroscopic surgery produces scarring and the subsequent inhibition of forward motion of the condyle. This inhibition is also caused by the secondary healing and contracture of the scar. The success rate after surgery was 93% for 120 joints in 75 patients with hypermobility. Fifty-five joints in 36 patients with recurrent dislocation were successfully treated over a 7-year period (32 after one operation and 4 after two procedures). Ohnishi[9] has also used the arthroscope to place a suture securing the posterior margin of the disk to the posterior wall of the capsule in order to inhibit forward sliding of the disk. Ohnishi's patients were placed in elastic intermaxillary traction for 2 or more weeks to limit opening.

In 1989, Qui and colleagues[10] compared the results of injecting a 5% sodium morrhuate solution into one side of the mandibular joint cavity of dogs with those of subsynovial injection into the opposite side. This was done using arthroscopy. Subsynovial injections were found to be more effective in producing scarring of the posterior disk attachment. Subsequently, utilizing arthroscopic control and local anesthesia, five patients with recurrent dislocation were treated with subsynovial injections in two or three areas of the posterior wall. Treatment was effective in all five patients, and there were no complications. This was a preliminary study, and the procedure was readily accepted by the patients.

METHODS

Arthroscopic mandibular joint surgery consisting of arthrolysis, lavage, manipulation, and sclerotherapy was completed in 95 joints for 53 patients. There were 9 males and 44 females, with a range in age from 15 to 76 years (mean age = 36). Thirty-seven patients (70%) had a significant history of macrotrauma. The duration of symptoms ranged from 6 months to 22 years, with an average duration of 5.5 years. There were 42 patients with hypermobility and 11 with recurrent mandibular dislocation. Eight of the patients with painful hypermobility had a history of mandibular dislocation. The patients were diagnosed with hypermobility based on radiographic and clinical evidence of condyle translation anterior to the articular eminence (Fig. 10–1), clinical evidence or a history of a wide range of mandibular motion, and the laxity of the disk and the capsule as observed during their arthroscopic diagnostic examinations. Wilkes'[11] method for the staging of internal derangement and an arthroscopic modification of this staging[12] were used (Tables 10–1 and 10–2). Staging was determined based on

patient history, physical examination, arthrotomography or magnetic resonance imaging, and on findings at arthroscopy. There were 24 patients in the early intermediate stage (stage II), 57 in the intermediate stage (stage III), 8 in the late intermediate stage (stage IV),

TABLE 10–1. WILKES' STAGING CLASSIFICATION FOR INTERNAL DERANGEMENT OF THE TEMPOROMANDIBULAR JOINT*

Stage I	(Early Stage) A. Clinical: No significant mechanical symptoms other than opening reciprocal clicking; no pain or limitation of motion. B. Radiologic: Slight forward displacement; good anatomic contour of the disk; negative tomograms. C. Anatomic/pathologic: Excellent anatomic form; slight anterior displacement; passive incoordination demonstrable.
Stage II	(Early/Intermediate Stage) A. Clinical: One or more episodes of pain; beginning major mechanical problems consisting of mid- to late-opening loud clicking, transient catching, and locking. B. Radiologic: Slight forward displacement; beginning disk deformity of slight thickening of posterior edge; negative tomograms. C. Anatomic/pathologic: Anterior disk displacement; early anatomic disk deformity; good central articulating area.
Stage III	(Intermediate Stage) A. Clinical: Multiple episodes of pain; major mechanical symptoms consisting of locking (intermittent or fully closed), restriction of motion, and difficulty with function. B. Radiologic: Anterior disk displacement with significant deformity/prolapse of disk (increased thickening of posterior edge); negative tomograms. C. Anatomic/pathologic: Marked anatomic disk deformity with anterior displacement; no hard tissue changes.
Stage IV	(Intermediate/Late Stage) A. Clinical: Slight increase in severity over intermediate stage. B. Radiologic: Increase in severity over intermediate stage; positive tomograms showing early to moderate degenerative changes (flattening of eminence, deformed condylar head, sclerosis). C. Anatomic/pathologic: Increase in severity over intermediate stage; hard tissue degenerative remodeling of both bearing surfaces (osteophytosis); multiple adhesions in anterior and posterior recesses; no perforation of disk or attachments.
Stage V	(Late Stage) A. Clinical: Characterized by crepitus, variable and episodic pain, chronic restriction of motion, and difficulty in function. B. Radiologic: Disk or attachment perforation; filling defects; gross anatomic deformity of disk and hard tissues; positive tomograms with essentially degenerative arthritic changes. C. Anatomic/pathologic: Gross degenerative changes of disk and hard tissues; perforation of posterior attachment; multiple adhesions; osteophytosis; flattening of condyle and eminence; subcortical cystic formation

*Wilkes, CH. Internal derangements of the temporomandibular joint. Arch Otolargynol Head Neck Surg (1989), 1:59–68.

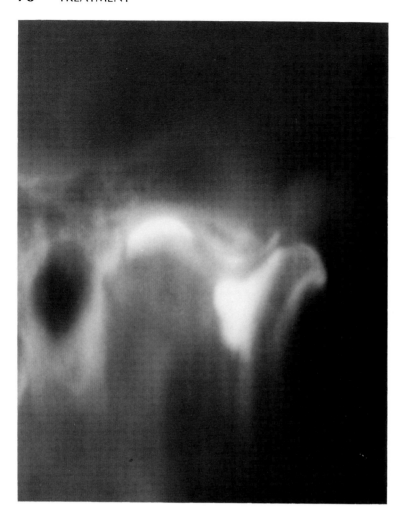

FIGURE 10–1. Dislocation of the condyle anterior and superior to the articular eminence and anterior to the disk. (From Qui, WL; Hu, G; Ha, G. Experimental Study and Preliminary Clinical Application of Subsynovial Sclerosing Injection Using an Arthroscope. Abstracts of the American Society of TMJ Surgeons Annual Meeting, Palm Springs, California, February 1989.)

and 6 in the late stage (stage V). The intermediate-stage patients had either a reducing disk or a chronic disk prolapse but maintained the ability to open their mouths wide. Frequently, the condyle would translate anterior to the dislocated and deformed disk. Subjective pain and dysfunction were present in all patients. Surgery was not performed unless signs and symptoms were associated with disability and nonsurgical care had failed to give satisfactory results. Internal derangement was present combined with the associated conditions of either hypermobility or recurrent dislocation.

All patients were treated surgically under general anesthesia that included a muscle relaxant. They were admitted and discharged from the hospital the same day. A physical examination to assess joint function and the range of mandibular motion was conducted while the patient was under general anesthesia prior to preparation and draping.

Transparent plastic drapes were placed in such a way so as to enable the assistant to manipulate the mandible intraorally. Such draping permitted either unilateral or bilateral procedures. It was possible to manipulate the mandible through the sterile drapes in order to facilitate diagnostic and surgical maneuvers. The assistant initially manipulated the mandible anteriorly to enable the surgeon to accurately palpate the preauricular pouch eminence, the condyle, and the lateral lip of the glenoid fossa. A pen was used to mark the skin to correspond to the location of the lateral lip and the eminence. This aided in the proper placement of puncture sites for single- or double-puncture techniques. The posterolateral puncture site of the fossa was used for diagnostic arthroscopy, and the anterolateral puncture site was used for the working cannula or for the spinal needle when performing triangulation techniques.

The arthroscopes used were either 1.9 mm or 2.7 mm in diameter. The cannulas used had outside diameters 0.4–0.7 mm greater than those of the scopes. A 2.7-mm diameter scope and its 3.4-mm diameter cannula were used for the majority of patients. The larger scope was used for single-puncture fossa procedures, whereas the smaller scope and cannulas were used for double-puncture techniques. A 19-gauge butterfly needle with tubing either attached or not attached to a source of suction was used for outflow. When using the larger scope, a small 3-mm vertical incision

TABLE 10–2. ARTHROSCOPIC STAGING OF INTERNAL JOINT DERANGEMENTS CORRELATED WITH WILKES' STAGING*

Stage I	(Early Stage) Characteristics: Roofing, 80% (closed position) to 100% (open or protrusive positions); incipient bilaminar zone elongation; normal disk flexure at the junction of discal eminence and the superior lamina; normal synovium; incipient loss of articular surface smoothness; normal superior compartment recesses and vascularity.
Stage II	(Early/Intermediate Stage) Characteristics: Roofing, 50% (closed) to 100% (open or protrusive); bilaminar elongation with decreased flexure; early adhesive synovitis with beginning adhesion formation; slight lateroanterior capsular prolapse.

Stage III	(Intermediate Stage)
	Characteristics: Advanced bilaminar elongation with accordion-shaped redundancy and loss of flexure; prominent synovitis; diminished lateral recess' advanced adhesion formations; anterior pseudowall formation in substage B.
	   Substage A: Roofing, 5% (closed) to <15% (open or protrusive); chondromalacia grades I–II (softening, blistering, or furrowing).
	   Substage B: No roofing; more severe anterior recess changes; chrondromalacia grades II–III (blistering, furrowing, ulceration, fraying, fibrillation, and surface rupture).

Stage IV	(Intermediate/Late Stage) Characteristics: Increase over intermediate stage disease; hyalinization of posterior attachment; chondromalacia grades III–IV (ulceration, fraying, furrowing, fibrillation, surface rupture, cratering, and bone exposure).
Stage V	(Late Stage) Characteristics: Prominent fibrillations on articular surfaces; perforation; retrodiscal hyalinization; false capsule formation anteriorly; generalized adhesions; advanced synovitis; chondromalacia grade IV (cratering and bone exposure).

*Bronstein, S. Arthroscopy: Historical perspectives and indications. Oral Maxillofac Surg Clin N Am (1989), 1:59–68.

was made in the preauricular pouch with a number 11 blade.

At the start of the procedure the mandible was retracted inferiorly and anteriorly by the assistant. This opened the joint and facilitated the insertion of a 22-gauge needle into the superior compartment from the inferolateral approach. Two to four milliliters of 0.5% bupivacaine hydrochloride with epinephrine 1:200,000 was injected to expand the superior joint space.

A systematic examination of the superior joint compartment was made after the cannulas, the scope, the camera, and the outflow tubing were in place. The assistant held the mandible in a forward and distracted position. The examination and the video recording started when the field of view was at the posterior attachment of the retrodiscal tissues to the fossa. The retrodiscal tissue was examined first from medial to lateral. Then the fossa was examined from lateral to medial. The medial capsule was examined along the medial paradiscal groove. The scope was then advanced in the posterior pouch from medial to lateral so that the posterior slope of the eminence and the posterior discal eminence (or retrodiscal tissue–eminence interface if the disk was displaced) could be observed. The lateral capsule, the lateral articular eminence disk, and the lateral paradiscal groove were viewed next. The scope was then placed near the entry point into the joint so that the motion and the position of the disk could be examined while the assistant gently seated the condyle in the fossa and moved the condyle–disk complex forward and back across the articular eminence. Catching, interference, and the degree of roofing of the condyle by the disk were observed. The condyle was then distracted and positioned forward. The scope was advanced to the medial wall and into the medial paradiscal groove. The condyle was manipulated posteriorly and distracted by applying pressure over the molars. The scope was moved from medial to lateral within the anterior synovial pouch in order to observe the capsule and the anterior discal tissues. Adhesions were often lysed when this maneuver was performed. Care was taken to avoid the scuffing of the fibrocartilage of the eminence. The scope was retracted again into the posterior pouch while the condyle was moved forward. The examination was then complete. Most adhesions were lysed by the sweeping movement of the scope and the cannula. The medial capsular wall and the oblique protuberance were identified once again. The cannula and the scope were placed over the oblique protuberance and held in position while the scope was removed and a blunt trocar placed into the cannula. The retrodiscal pad was then retracted by manipulating the trocar posteriorly and inferiorly. The assistant simultaneously manipulated the mandible inferiorly, anteriorly, and to the opposite side of the displaced disk. Disk deformity may not allow the disk to be reduced; however, recently locked disks without deformity were reduced into an improved condyle–disk relationship. The disk-eminence interface and the degree of roofing of the disk during motion of the condyle were examined once again. With the condyle in a forward position the posterior band of the disk was visible at the interface. If the disk had been successfully reduced the band remained in this position during anterior and posterior movement of the condyle. The joint was continually lavaged with lactated Ringer's solution.

The most frequently employed method for the subsynovial injection of the sclerosant into the oblique protuberance area was triangulation of a 12-cm, 18-gauge spinal needle without a cannula (Fig. 10–2). A custom-made working scope was occasionally used (Fig. 10–3). This scope was made by soldering an 18-gauge spinal needle to the cannula for the 1.9-mm scope. This facilitated placement of a 20-gauge, 16-cm

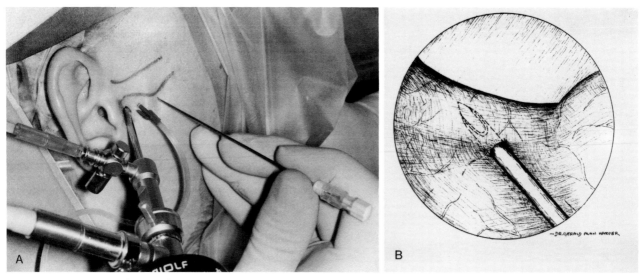

FIGURE 10–2. *A*—Triangulation technique using a spinal needle for the subsynovial injection of sclerosant. A 25-degree 2.7-mm diameter arthroscope is positioned in the posterior portal to view the oblique protuberance. The spinal needle is inserted through an anterior portal slightly anterior and inferior to the articular tubercle of the eminence. *B*—Drawing of an arthroscopic view of the right posterior superior synovial pouch. The spinal needle is inserted into the subsynovial tissue of the posterior disk attachment near or in the oblique protuberance under direct vision. (From Merrill, RG. Mandibular dislocation and hypermobility. Oral Maxillofac Surg Clin N Am (1989), 1:399–413.)

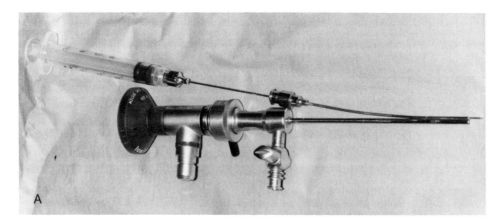

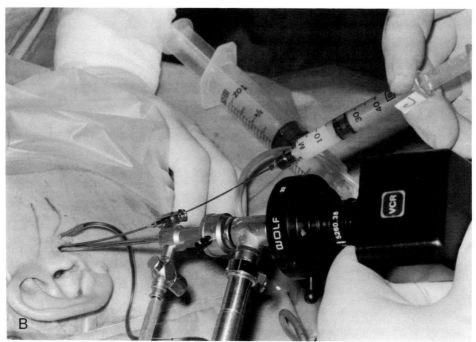

FIGURE 10–3. *A*—A custom-made working scope with an 18-gauge spinal needle soldered to the cannula of a 1.9-mm scope. *B*—A 20-gauge spinal needle is placed through the 18-gauge needle for injection into the oblique protuberance under direct vision.

spinal needle via the soldered 18-gauge needle into the direct view of the 25-degree scope and into the oblique protuberance. Triangulation using an anterior working cannula was also employed for sclerotherapy after the completion of arthrolysis, lavage, and manipulation. A 20-gauge spinal needle 16 cm in length was inserted through the anterior working cannula and directed into the oblique protuberance under direct vision. One-half milliliter of a 1% sodium tetradecyl sulfate solution (5 mg) was injected into the joints of patients with painful hypermobility, and 1 ml of a 3% solution of the same (30 mg) was injected into the 11 joints of patients with recurrent dislocation. This was followed by the injection of 1 ml of 0.5% bupivacaine hydrochloride with 1:200,000 epinephrine. The joint was again lavaged with lactated Ringer's solution before the removal of instruments and the one-suture closure of the puncture site.

Postoperative care for patients with hypermobility and recurrent dislocation included limited motion of the mandible. The patients with recurrent dislocation were placed in maxillomandibular elastic fixation for 4 weeks. After this period a soft diet requiring no chewing was started and continued for at least 2 months. A moderate range of motion exercise commenced after the release of fixation. An occlusal appliance was used in bruxism patients if occlusal treatment was part of their comprehensive treatment plan. The patients with hypermobility were not placed in maxillomandibular fixation but were instructed to limit their mouth opening to no greater than 25 mm. Several exercises designed to open the mouth 25 mm four times a day were recommended. Wide opening and yawning were avoided or restricted, and the patients were placed on a soft diet for 3 months. The medications used were a narcotic analgesic (for the first few postoperative days) and a nonsteroidal antiinflammatory drug (for 2 weeks). For those with significant myofascial components to their disorders a muscle relaxant was prescribed. Work and activities that would place the joint at risk for injury were avoided.

RESULTS

The patients were evaluated based on a physical examination and a questionnaire developed by Dolwick and Nitzen[13] (Fig. 10–4). Forty-eight joints were found to have improved, 5 showed no change, and none were worse, resulting in a 91% success rate. The success rate correlated to the diagnosis of each joint as follows: 22 joints in stage II were improved and 2 remained the same; 55 joints in stage III showed improvement and 2 remained the same; 5 in stage IV were improved and 3 stayed the same; and 5 in stage V showed improvement and 1 remained the same. No joints or

TABLE 10–3. RESULTS OF SCLEROTHERAPY AND LLM* FOR 53 PATIENTS (95 JOINTS)

Number of Patients	Number of Patients Showing Improvement	Number of Patients Showing No Improvement
53	48 (91%)	5 (9%)

*Lysis, lavage, and manipulation.

patients were worse after surgery. The results of lysis, lavage, and manipulation with sclerotherapy as compared with those of a similar group of 98 patients who received the same treatment without sclerotherapy are shown in Tables 10–3 to 10–6. The most impressive improvement with the addition of sclerotherapy was seen in displaced disks that would reduce on opening. In particular, stage II internal derangement and intermediate stage III disks with definite deformity of their posterior band would improve. The success rate was 91% among stage II internal derangement patients who underwent sclerotherapy and 65% for those who did not. For stage III patients the success rates were 96% and 85%, respectively. There were no complications in patients who underwent lysis, lavage, and manipulation combined with chemical sclerotherapy. There were also no instances of recurrent dislocation. The range of mandibular motion was not excessively limited by sclerotherapy and was maintained within normal limits.

DISCUSSION

A serious effort to evaluate the effectiveness of arthroscopic diagnostic and operative procedures used in the treatment of pathologic conditions of the TMJ has been made since 1985. The procedure of arthroscopic lysis, lavage, and disk manipulation is a form of arthroplasty. It is applied as the first surgical option for patients with internal derangements who present with indications for arthrotomy. The indications include an accurate diagnosis of internal derangement or other arthropathy, which is the source of a patient's debilitating signs and symptoms, and the condition that nonsurgical therapies have been unsuccessful. After 3 years of using arthroscopic lysis, lavage, and manipu-

TABLE 10–4. RESULTS OF LLM* FOR 98 PATIENTS (157 JOINTS)

Number of Patients	Number of Patients Showing Improvement	Number of Patients Showing No Improvement
98	76 (78%)	35 (22%)

*Lysis, lavage, and manipulation.

NAME _____

DATE _____

PLEASE CIRCLE THE CORRECT RESPONSE WHERE INDICATED:

1. Do you have any pain now?   YES   NO
   If YES, please answer questions 2 and 3, if NO please go to question 4.

2. Please rate your pain by placing an "X" on the line indicating (A) your present pain and (B) your usual pain. Mark each "X" with the corresponding letter:

_____

NO PAIN   MOST INTENSE PAIN IMAGINABLE

3. Please indicate on the drawing those areas where you have pain.

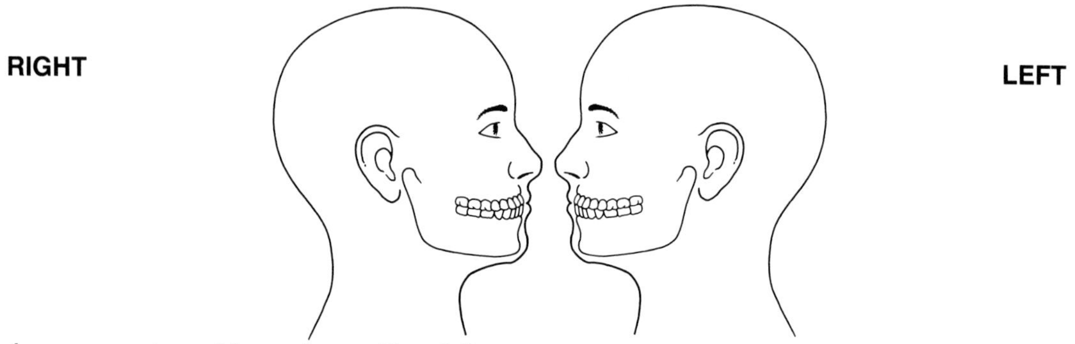

RIGHT   **LEFT**

4. Are you awakened from sleep with pain?   YES   NO
5. Are you aware of clenching or grinding of your teeth?   YES   NO
6. Is the pain worse on functioning (chewing, talking)?   YES   NO
7. Do you have limited opening?   YES   NO
8. Do you have any dietary limitation related to your jaw problem? YES   NO
9. Does your jaw make noises on functioning?   YES   NO
10. Have you experienced jaw locking since the treatment?   YES   NO
11. How do you feel now compared to the time you were treated here?

_____

WORSE   ORIGINALLY   BETTER

12. Please rate your ability to chew by placing an "X" on the line indicating your present ability to chew.

_____

NO DIFFICULTY CHEWING   UNABLE TO CHEW

13. How can you chew now compared to when you were treated here?

_____

WORSE   ORIGINALLY   BETTER

14. Please indicate if you will return for an examination.   YES   NO

FIGURE 10–4. Follow-up evaluation form. (Courtesy of F. Dolwick and D. Nitzen.)

TABLE 10–5. RESULTS OF SCLEROTHERAPY AND LLM* AS A FUNCTION OF DIAGNOSIS IN 53 PATIENTS (95 JOINTS)

Stage of Internal Derangement	Number of Joints Showing Improvement	Number of Joints Showing No Improvement
II	22 (91%)	2 (9%)
III	55 (96%)	2 (4%)
IV	5 (63%)	3 (37%)
V	5 (83%)	1 (17%)

*Lysis, lavage, and manipulation.

lation the results were sufficiently positive to continue its use as a first surgical option. Arthrotomy procedures continued to be performed for patients who underwent unsuccessful arthroscopic surgery and for patients with ankylosis, tumors, condylar loss, and implant arthropathy.

For patients with recurrent dislocation, the treatment of the posterior disk attachment by subsynovial chemical injection in the area of the oblique protuberance was initiated in late 1987. The results of the treatment of this disorder were impressive with respect not only to the elimination of dislocations but also in the significant reduction or elimination of pain. Later, in 1988, the technique was applied in the treatment of patients with painful internal derangements and hypermobility. The results were equally satisfying in this group of patients. Not one complication occurred and no patient required a repeat arthroscopic or arthrotomy procedure. This is significant compared with results obtained by those surgeons who advocated a series of two to three injections of stronger sodium psylliate or sodium morrhuate sclerosing solutions directly into the joint cavity. The arthroscopic procedure of lysis, lavage, and manipulation without sclerotherapy for patients with painful hypermobility and stage II internal derangement had the highest failure rate as compared with the treatment of other stages of internal derangement. It was this category that most often required arthrotomy and disk repair after failed arthroscopy, usually in the first 9 months after the arthroscopic procedure. The addition of chemical sclerotherapy to the arthroscopic lysis, lavage, and manipulation procedure improved treatment results. It is an accurate, safe, and conservative surgical treatment for patients having either symptomatic hypermobility or recurrent mandibular dislocation. A difference between the two groups that may affect their accurate comparison was that the lysis, lavage, and manipulation group without sclerotherapy had a 4-year follow-up, whereas the group receiving sclerotherapy had a 1- to 2-year follow-up.

Lysis, lavage, and manipulation for the treatment of internal derangement patients without hypermobility and the same procedure in combination with chemical sclerotherapy in the treatment of patients with internal derangement, hypermobility, and recurrent mandibular dislocation were found to have satisfactory results. The results compare well with those of arthrotomy procedures for the same conditions; therefore, the more conservative arthroscopic surgery offers an attractive alternative to arthrotomy procedures.

Mandibular hypermobility in association with derangement of the disk is quite common. It is probable that hypermobile joints become symptomatic as a result of trauma. Many methods of treatment are only partially successful for the group of patients with this disorder. The addition of sclerotherapy to arthroscopic surgery is a significant improvement in the treatment of these patients. Arthroscopic lysis, lavage, and manipulation offers the advantages of improved disk mobility and position prior to the accurate subsynovial injection of a small amount of sclerosant under direct vision via the scope. The sclerosant most likely produces its effect by causing tissue irritation and fibroblastic activity.

SUMMARY

An application of sclerotherapy for painful hypermobility and recurrent mandibular dislocation involves the injection of the mild sclerosant sodium tetradecylsulfate into the posterior disk attachment by arthroscopic technique. One injection of 1 ml of a 1–3% solution followed by 3–4 weeks of limited mouth opening has proved to be satisfactory. The application of arthroscopic arthrocentesis and intraarticular manipulations to lyse adhesions and reposition amenable disks is performed first. The use of triangulation for direct visualization enables one to accurately inject the sclerosant into the subsynovial tissues of the posterior disk attachment. Results have been impressive not only in eliminating dislocations but also in alleviating pain. This technique is a viable alternative to the various arthrotomy procedures when a surgical approach is indicated.

TABLE 10–6. RESULTS OF LLM* AS A FUNCTION OF DIAGNOSIS IN 98 PATIENTS (157 JOINTS)

Stage of Internal Derangement	Number of Joints Showing Improvement	Number of Joints Showing No Improvement
II	22 (65%)	12 (35%)
III	65 (85%)	12 (15%)
IV	21 (80%)	5 (20%)
V	13 (67%)	7 (33%)

*Lysis, lavage, and manipulation.

REFERENCES

1. Schultz, LW. A treatment for subluxation of the temporomandibular joint. JAMA (1937), 109:1032.
2. Schultz, LW. Report of ten years' experience in treating hypermobility of the temporomandibular joint. J Oral Surg (1947), 5:202–207.
3. Schultz, LW; Shriner, W. Treatment of acute and chronic temporomandibular joint arthritis. J Fla Med Assoc (1943), 30:189.
4. Moose, SM. Experimental injections of fibrosing solutions into the temporomandibular joints of monkeys. J Am Dent Assoc (1941), 28:761–765.
5. McKelvy, LE. Sclerosing solution in the treatment of chronic subluxation of the temporomandibular joint. J Oral Surg (1950), 8:225.
6. Thoma, KH. Textbook of Oral Surgery. (3rd Ed.) St. Louis: CV Mosby Co. (1958), 724–727.
7. Archer, WH. Survey of mandibular joint injection with sclerosing solution. Lecture presented to the Great Lakes Society of Oral Surgeons, Chicago, Illinois, May 1975.
8. Ohnishi, M; Nakayama, E; Kino, K. Arthroscopic surgery for habitual dislocations of the temporomandibular joint [Japanese]. Arthroscopy (1987), 12:103–105.
9. Ohnishi, M. Arthroscopic surgery for hypermobility and recurrent mandibular dislocation. Oral Maxillofac Surg Clin N Am (1989), 1:153–164.
10. Qui, WL; Hu, G; Ha, G. Experimental study and preliminary clinical application of subsynovial sclerosing injection using an arthroscope. Abstracts of the American Society of TMJ Surgeons Annual Meeting, Palm Springs, California, February 1989.
11. Wilkes, CH. Internal derangements of the temporomandibular joint. Arch Otolaryngol Head Neck Surg (1989), 115:469–477.
12. Bronstein, S. Arthroscopy: Historical perspectives and indications. Oral Maxillofac Surg Clin N Am (1989), 1:59–68.
13. Dolwick, F; Nitzen, D. Personal communication, 1988.

Eleven

Arthroscopic Treatment of the Human Temporomandibular Joint

GLENN T. CLARK, D.D.S., M.S.
CHANGRUI LIU, D.D.S.

Even though the first recorded arthroscopic procedure on a human was performed by Takagi in 1918[1] the temporomandibular joint (TMJ) was not probed with an arthroscopic instrument until 1975.[2] The early TMJ arthroscopic forays were primarily diagnostic endeavors,[3-19] but surgical applications soon followed.[1,16,18,20-35] The primary disease addressed by arthroscopic surgeons has been TMJ internal derangement, especially the condition described as anteriorly displaced disk without reduction.[2,31,34,36] Judged solely on the basis of the growing number of articles and books being published on TMJ arthroscopic surgery, it appears that this procedure has gained widespread acceptance as a clinically effective method of treatment. Unfortunately, there is a paucity of random-assignment, controlled, and scientifically sound clinical trials upon which to base the acceptance of arthroscopic surgeries as a substitute for more traditional, nonsurgical and surgical approaches. This chapter critically reviews the existing literature and examines the reasons for acceptance of arthroscopic surgical techniques.

DIAGNOSTIC ARTHROSCOPY IN THE HUMAN TMJ

As in other joints, arthroscopy provides valuable diagnostic information about the intraarticular structures of the TMJ that cannot be obtained with other methods.[37] Imaging methods, such as temporomandib-

ular arthrography, computed tomography (CT), and magnetic resonance imaging (MRI), provide a two-dimensional, static image of the TMJ.[36] Three-dimensional reconstruction of the TMJ using MRI images has begun to be performed. However, unlike two-dimensional and three-dimensional imaging, arthroscopy provides a direct and detailed view of the actual surfaces of the joint and the disk. An important question is, Which suspected TMJ diseases or disorders are the best candidates for these various diagnostic imaging procedures and, in the case of diagnostic arthroscopy, for direct visualization?

Several research reports have appeared that address this question. In 1989 Bibb and colleagues conducted a cadaver study comparing the diagnostic strengths and limitations of arthroscopy with those of arthrography and tomography.[19] They reported that the soft tissue morphology represented in subsequent dissections was not completely discovered by any of the imaging procedures evaluated in their study. They also reported that the posterior fibrous limits of the disk could not be determined from the silhouette of the disk seen in an arthrogram. A partial explanation for these results is the fact that the contours of the bone tissue, observed using radiographic imaging methods, and those of soft tissue, observed using arthroscopy, are not predictably congruent.[38,39] Furthermore, the assumed disk landmark of a posterior inferior bulge commonly described in an arthrogram is based on the assumption that the disk still has a biconcave shape. As this assumption is not uniformly correct, many judgments on disk position are potentially incorrect. The article by Bibb and colleagues did not address how accurately an arthroscopic examination was able to determine disk position.

The diagnostic accuracy of TMJ arthroscopy has also been investigated in rabbits,[3,40] in cadaver material,[8,12,19,41] and in human patients.[14] Contradictory results have emerged among these studies. For example, in 1985 Holmlund and Hellsing[8] reported an accuracy rate of 100% for the arthroscopic diagnosis of arthrosis; in other studies the rates of accurate arthrosis detection were much lower.[12-19]

Data on the accuracy of arthroscopy for the diagnosis of adhesions were not included in early studies[8,12] because the significance of adhesions was not recognized until later. Sanders[20] described synovial adhesions in patients with nonreducing anterior disk displacement. The adhesions were most commonly located in the posterior recess, from the posterior slope of the eminence to the central portion of the disk.

To assess the accuracy of the arthroscopic diagnosis of perforations and adhesions, a study on 28 fresh cadavers was performed to evaluate the presence of disk perforations and adhesions within the TMJ upper compartment.[41] The findings from arthroscopy were compared with those recorded at subsequent dissection. The results suggested that an arthroscopic diagnosis of perforations is reasonably reliable; however, arthroscopy was not found to be successful in the diagnosis of perforations. This conclusion was based on the fact that two thirds of the perforations identified at dissection were not visualized arthroscopically. These results actually confirm the results of a smaller study performed by Liedberg and Westesson.[12] In their research, the number of accurate arthroscopic diagnoses of adhesions was greater than that for perforations (three of four joints with adhesions were identified correctly).

The most common location of perforations—in the lateral and medial fields—may make their identification during arthroscopy difficult when using the lateral entry approach. The lateral puncture site does not permit good visualization of the most lateral part of the joint. From a diagnostic perspective these limitations are unfortunate because the lateral third has been reported to have the highest incidence of osteoarthrosis,[42-44] deviation in form,[43,45] and disk thinning.[46] The radiographic imaging of the lateral condylar third was also frequently less than ideal because of the rapidly changing rate of contour.[19] Arthroscopy is not the only technique that presents problems in detecting perforations. MRI frequently fails to detect perforations, and fluoroarthroscopy has been known to produce iatrogenic perforations.

Another difficult area to view during arthroscopy in cadavers[41] and in patients[47] is the anterior recess of the upper joint compartment. An additional puncture site or the use of a different type of optics may overcome this problem.

It has been claimed that arthroscopy can determine a disk's position in a joint. In fact, specific arthroscopic criteria on the basis of which a disk displacement can be judged were offered by Blaustein and Heffez in 1988.[15] The validity of these criteria has not yet been tested. However, many specialists have speculated that although these criteria aid in the recognition of a grossly displaced disk they are less helpful in making finite judgments of less severe disk position abnormalities as it is usually difficult to differentiate the remodeled retrodiscal tissue from the remodeled posterior band, even in histologic sections. In addition, the disk and condyle are not necessarily in a normal position after the infusion of fluid during the procedure. Finally, arthroscopy provides only a narrow perspective of the superficial tissues and does not show the underlying bone (the landmark used for making positional determination).

Arthroscopic surgeons occasionally report the presence of hyperplastic or hyperemic tissues in the TMJ. Before such an observation can be significant, however, the criteria for determining the presence of such tissues must be tested and the range of normal joint tissue appearance must be better explored. Furthermore, the clinical significance of hyperplastic and hyperemic soft tissue is not yet known.[41]

Osteoarthrosis (OA) is considered a primarily noninflammatory degenerative joint disease, and OA of the TMJ has been extensively investigated in autopsy studies.[43,44,48-52] An arthroscopic examination of 42 joints for the presence and location of OA and synovitis in the superior TMJ has been reported.[53] The study showed that OA was present in 74% of the joints, and the predominant location of the OA was the posterior slope of the eminence. The investigators reported that the disk was not usually affected, but when it was, changes in the laterocentral part of the disk were seen. Furthermore, synovitis was found to occur in 52% of the joints.

To summarize, there have been many claims on the diagnostic value of arthroscopy but few actual controlled experiments to test these claims. Most of the studies that have been undertaken utilized small numbers of old cadaver specimens. Also, many of the prior studies were largely preliminary in nature and often defined untested criteria for abnormality as a part of the analysis. It is clear that an additional series of well-designed, comparative diagnostic methodology studies are still needed. These studies will need to define the specific conditions being evaluated and, specifically, the stage of the condition at which the use of a particular diagnostic method is appropriate.

CLASSIFICATION SCHEMES FOR ARTHROSCOPIC NOMENCLATURE

The arthroscopic nomenclature scheme introduced in 1981 has not been widely used, possibly because it does not lend itself easily to the communication and the description of normal, pathologic, and postsurgical findings.[54,55] A revision of this scheme that better describes the anterior and posterior synovial pouches was reported in 1985.[56] This improved classification scheme described regions above and below the disk without regard to stable references. A competing regional anatomic nomenclature and arthroscopic terminology scheme based on osseous landmarks was introduced in 1987.[13] This scheme subdivides the upper space into a posterior (or glenoid) region and an anterior (or preeminence) region. The apex of the articular eminence serves as the boundary for these two regions. It has yet to be determined which scheme will achieve widespread acceptance.

SURGICAL ARTHROSCOPY OF THE TMJ

A frequently stated advantage of arthroscopy is that it not only assists in diagnosis but also facilitates direct surgical intervention. Conventional wisdom dictates that most patients with TMJ disease or dysfunction undergo a course of nonsurgical treatment (usually including occlusal appliance use, diet restrictions, nonsteroidal antiinflammatory agents, muscle relaxants, physical therapy, and psychologic management) prior to any surgical therapy, including arthroscopy. Based on a review of the literature, it is obvious that arthroscopy is being used more and more frequently as a form of intervention. This change in sequencing is largely due to the fact that arthroscopy is generally well tolerated by patients and rarely results in complications.

Indications for Surgical Arthroscopy

Arthroscopy is a surgical procedure and therefore must only be selected when the indications are very clear. The literature has described the presence of the following conditions as indications for the technique: disk displacement with reduction and pain, disk displacement without reduction, intraarticular adhesion disorders, rheumatoid arthritis, postsurgical adhesions and TMJ hypomobility.[36] It is also indicated for the diagnosis of local tumor invasion into the TMJ, synovitis,[57] hypermobility,[30,35,57] recurrent mandibular dislocation,[30] and when joint tissue biopsy is needed.

Although arthroscopy can be implemented for the treatment of a large number of conditions, data on the therapeutic effectiveness of arthroscopy for each problem are very limited. Because some of the conditions described have quite divergent levels of symptom presentation, it is essential to be certain that a patient's primary pain and dysfunction is of an articular origin. Diagnostic intraarticular anesthetic blockade may be required to confirm this. The literature generally supports the view that surgery should never be undertaken in any patient whose disability is minor and nonprogressive. Appropriate nonsurgical therapy should precede any surgical intervention. Nonsurgical therapy should include not only the usual and customary physical medicine and the use of occlusal appliances but also behavioral medicine, such as stress management. Surgical therapy is not likely to be effective when a patient's pain is related to a nonarticular disorder such as myofascial pain.[57]

Contraindications to Arthroscopy

There are several basic contraindications to arthroscopy described in the literature. They include obesity (where it is not possible to adequately palpate the joint space), any TMJ or ear infection, skin infections (such as acne in the region over the TMJ,[36] severe bony or fibrous ankylosis with marked impairment of joint mobility,[37] and any metastatic or malignant tumor owing to possible tumor seeding.[57]

Anesthetic Considerations During TMJ Arthroscopy

General anesthesia with nasal tracheal intubation is most commonly employed when arthroscopic diagnosis and surgery are performed.* However, there are several reports in the literature describing arthroscopy performed in patients under local anesthesia.[13,37,47,58] Whereas arthroscopy in patients under general anesthesia allows more vigorous exploration and therapy, local anesthesia is advantageous in that the patient can participate in assessing the procedure's effect on functional ability. In order to achieve efficient local anesthesia, the auriculotemporal nerve must be blocked at a location posterior to the condylar neck. This usually involves infiltrating the nerve approximately 3 ml of lidocaine with epinephrine (10 mg/ml).[37] Most arthroscopic surgical procedures are performed in patients under general anesthesia; arthroscopy in patients under local anesthesia has been limited primarily to diagnostic forays.

---

*See references 1, 7, 16, 23, 26, 30, and 36.

Preauricular Anatomy and TMJ Arthroscopic Surgical Approaches

Absolute knowledge of the normal and atypical anatomy of the surgical site is essential with any invasive procedure. The location of important anatomic structures in the preauricular area has been described in various ways.[1,13,17,37,59–73]

The temporomandibular disk divides the joint into a superior and an inferior compartment. When distended, the superior compartment has a volume of approximately 2 ml, whereas the volume of the inferior compartment is only 1 ml. The exterior or lateral capsule is fibrous and therefore mildly resistant to puncture by an instrument. The disk–condyle complex is drawn forward with the condyle and simultaneously rotates around to the back side of the condyle during opening. This forward translation leaves a vacated temporomandibular fossa that is clearly palpable.[37]

This vacated region makes the superior joint space readily accessible. It is probably no coincidence that the most common and widely used TMJ arthroscopic approach is entry through the superior joint space. Some surgeons advocate that entry from a posterolateral direction is the best method to avoid contact with vital anatomic structures, such as arteries and nerves, that surround the TMJ.[36] In fact, Greene and colleagues[72] examined the relationships between arthroscopic surgery and the TMJ region in 36 cadavers. They reported that the maxillary artery and the main bifurcation of the facial nerve are located at a safe distance from the usual lateral arthroscopic approach to the TMJ. Their findings were: (1) the facial nerve frontal branch was typically found 3 mm or more anterior to the midpoint of the lateral pole of the condyle; (2) the superficial temporal vessels and the auriculotemporal nerve were frequently very close to puncture sites; (3) the bony floor of the glenoid fossa had an average thickness of 0.9 mm; and (4) the external soft tissue auditory canal traveled in a somewhat anterior direction, thereby necessitating a skin puncture perpendicular to the bony canal approximately 7 mm anterior to the posterior aspect of the tragus. Unfortunately, the TMJ compartment approaches compared were not described by Greene and colleagues in detail.

In another cadaver study, the best puncture site was described to be 10–13 mm from the most central and posterior aspect of the tragus on the tragal–lateral canthus line.[8] An alternative is puncturing approximately 5–7 mm below the inferior border of the zygomatic arch.[16]

This entry site is by no means the only acceptable method. In fact, there are five joint entry approaches described in the literature: (1) the superior postero-lateral approach,[13,15,17,36,58,68] (2) the superior anterolateral approach,[68] (3) the inferior posterolateral approach,[58,68,74] (4) the inferior anterolateral approach,[68,74] and (5) the endaural approach.[68,75–77]

Arthroscopic Treatment Results

Arthroscopy has become an alternative to open surgical arthrotomy for the treatment of certain conditions involving the TMJ. It has been reported to be very effective in eliminating symptoms of TMJ pain and especially for the management of acute, subacute, and sometimes even chronic limitations of movement of this joint.[34] The data from several studies of arthroscopic surgery can be combined to produce a demographic representation of the patients who have undergone this procedure. Patients ranged in age from 9 to 68 years, and follow-up was typically 24 months, with a range of 1 to 37 months.* The female-to-male ratio ranged from 6:1 to 8:1;[17,24,29,35] 51.1% of the patients received bilateral procedures, whereas 48.9% received unilateral procedures.[67] No random controlled research has been performed to evaluate the enthusiastic claims of success made in these reports. These claims and the existing literature are reviewed in detail later in this chapter.

Arthroscopic Treatment of Disk Displacement Without Reduction

Restricted translation of the mandibular condyle is a condition that can result from some combination of disk perforation, condyle and disk deformation, disk and articular surface adherence, or disk displacement without reduction.[78,79] Treatment alternatives to the nonsurgical approach have included open TMJ surgery (diskectomy and discoplasty), which may help decrease pain but frequently results in a chronic, partial restriction of jaw motion. Arthroscopy is an attractive alternative because it is less invasive than open surgery and is potentially more definitive than the symptomatic management of a restricted joint.[34]

Published studies have largely shown the clinical success of arthroscopic surgery as a treatment modality, reporting significant improvement in 80–92% of patients. Patients who underwent arthroscopy generally experienced a substantial reduction in pain.[1,20,23,27,28,67] Most of these studies reported a substantial improvement in jaw functional ability as a result of arthroscopy. In a clinical report evaluating 237 patients' postarthroscopic surgery, 63% of the patients had an increase in

*See references 10, 23, 24, 26, 27, 29, 34, and 35.

opening 1 month after surgery, 52% of whom displayed an increase in opening of more than 5 mm.[29] After 1 year 73% of the patients had an interincisal opening of 40 mm or greater. One report observed that the patients who had the most improvement in mobility were those who started with a restricted opening of 30 mm or less.[24] The mean increase in opening for these patients was 11.4 mm immediately following arthroscopy. These data might appear impressive at first glance, but it should be remembered that many patients have a substantial improvement in the severity of their symptoms within 6 months even without surgery.

For those whose symptoms do not change or worsen by the end of the first postoperative month, further significant improvement may not occur. It has been suggested that these patients should be considered for arthrotomic procedures to be performed after a waiting period of 6 to 12 months.[24]

The reports discussed are largely descriptive methodologic articles or retrospective case reviews compiled by surgeons themselves. Such case reviews provide valuable initial data about a new procedure, but are subject to bias and may not yield a careful evaluation of the procedure. The weight of the reported evidence does not lie in the quality of the research because no truly controlled, blind study has yet been performed. The primary strength of these open clinical trials is the similarity of their reported treatment results. Obviously, what is now needed is a random-assignment comparison study of treatment.

A Prospective Study of Long-term Outcome

Although they did not perform a controlled or randomized clinical trial, Clark and associates published the results of a prospective 2-year study of treatment outcome for 18 arthroscopy patients.[34] These patients had been treated using arthroscopic lysis and lavage of the superior compartment. All data were collected in a clinical research center by an independent examiner. The subjects' mean pain score at the final assessment had decreased by 57%. Jaw function showed an average improvement of 67%, and maximum active opening ability showed a 13-mm mean increase. Jaw joint clicking noises were slightly increased after arthroscopic surgery. The remarkable long-term success of arthroscopic surgery and the reduced morbidity and minimal invasiveness of the technique suggest that the mechanism of reduced condyle translation may be due in part to disk eminence adherence. This assumption is based on the increased mobility observed after arthroscopy, even though the disk was not reduced by the procedure. In other words,

physical blockage of condylar movement due to disk displacement does not fully explain the hypomobility seen in patients with closed-lock. The results strongly suggest that arthroscopy may be an effective therapy for a majority of patients with closed-lock and that therapeutic concern about disk position is overemphasized.

Disk Position After Arthroscopy

Gabler and coworkers published a study in which they used MRI to assess disk-condyle relationships before and after arthroscopic surgery.[28] No significant differences in the joint space in the closed position were found among control, prearthroscopic, and postarthroscopic treatment groups. Disk–condyle distance relationships in the open and the closed positions as measured using MRI did not significantly change after arthroscopic treatment. Another study utilized arthrography to assess discal position immediately following the arthroscopic manipulation of discal tissue.[80] Fourteen of 15 joints showed no evidence of improvement in discal position after arthroscopic surgery. These results are in agreement with those found in other reports in the literature.[1,26] The findings suggest that disk repositioning may not be necessary in order to achieve clinical success.

Joint Improvement After Arthroscopy

Two independent studies have reported no significant improvement in the incidence of joint sounds following arthroscopy.[26,34] Furthermore, even though the basic form and the position of the disk are not changed, factors indicating the success of arthroscopic surgery include both decreased pain and increased mobility. The pain relief is likely due to inflammatory substances within the joint, which are reduced postoperatively as a result of the lavage and the steroid injection. The increased joint mobility is probably related to a combination of tissue stretching and the release of abnormal intraarticular restraints (adhesions) that cause capsular strain. Other possible explanations for symptom improvement may be the effect of the postoperative bite appliance or the physical therapy, or both.[1,81]

Complications of TMJ Arthroscopy

Several complications resulting from TMJ arthroscopic procedures have been reported, and the number of reports of such complications has paralleled the increasing number of published articles on TMJ arthroscopy. Complications include infection,[20] hemorrhage,[10,13,36] sensory and motor nerve injury,[13] damage to the synovium of the joint or to the articular surfaces or the disk, or both,[17,36,82] persistent pain and swelling,[10] damage to the middle ear[82] and the middle cranial fossa,[17] instrument breakage in the joint,[31] and recurrent fibrous adhesions.[35] The risk of postoperative infection seems very low,[10,23,47,53] although a single case of postoperative infection has been reported.[20]

In comparison with the outcome of open TMJ surgical procedures, there are few peri- and postoperative complications following arthroscopic surgery,[10,17,20,23,47,53] especially when performed by an experienced surgeon.[23]

Disk Suturing Procedures

The literature clearly indicates that it is quite difficult, if not impossible, to alter discal position by the standard methods used in arthroscopic lavage and lysis surgery. No well-designed and controlled study has yet been performed that shows any long-term change in disk position as a result of surgical arthroscopy of any kind. The disk appears to always return to its original position as dictated by the bony confines into which it fits. Several new techniques that claim to return the disk to a more normal position have been advanced. These techniques claim to achieve disk position changes by fixing the disk with one or two sutures that are passed through the discal tissues and tied posteriorly, usually in the external auditory meatus.[25,31,35,83] In the first few days after surgery the disk is vulnerable to redisplacement during postoperative events such as vomiting, coughing, yawning, and sneezing, or after injury.[31]

Arthroscopic Suture with Cautery Treatment

To further aid in maintaining the disk in the new position, surgeons have attempted to combine the suturing technique with the scarification of intraarticular tissues by cautery.[31,35] This is performed by passing an electrosurgery instrument through an arthroscopic cannula. Continuous high-flow irrigation is applied while the target tissue (usually the posterior ligament) is cauterized. In theory, scarring and subsequent constriction of the posterior attachment will occur without long-term damage to the synovial tissues or to the ligament. Whether the disk will subsequently move to and remain in a more suitable position has yet to be proved.

Outcome Reports of Treatment Incorporating Suture, Cautery, or Laser Scarification

Tarro conducted an uncontrolled, open clinical trial in which 40 TMJs were treated using the suturing technique.[31] Fourteen of these joints received a combination of suture and cauterization of the posterior attachment. Successful results, defined as the restoration of normal jaw function without pain and an absence of joint noises, were observed in 36 joints. The postsurgical observation period ranged from 2 to 12 months, and no complications were reported. Unfortunately, however, the study defined neither the criteria used for diagnosis nor how treatment success was judged.[31,35]

In another open clinical trial without controls or defined criteria for measuring outcome, good clinical results were reported for 120 joints undergoing surgery in 75 patients with hypermobility.[30] Specifically, the author reported that 93% of the treatments for hypermobility were judged to be "markedly effective" or "effective." This same study also reported on 55 surgically treated joints in 36 patients with recurrent mandibular dislocation. Twenty-four of the joints in 12 of the patients achieved good clinical results (no dislocation recurred). All cases were treated by arthroscopic laser and disk suturing.

The Need for Further Research in TMJ Arthroscopy

The reports on surgical treatments for internal derangement of the TMJ (i.e., reconstructive arthroplasty, disk repositioning, meniscus repair, and eminectomy) indicate a postsurgical no-improvement and failure rate of 2–15%.[84–90] Unfortunately, these reports are all open and uncontrolled clinical case descriptions often without specific success criteria. Even so, these data imply that open surgical procedures for the treatment of internal derangement of the TMJ have been reasonably successful. Overall, comparable success has been reported for arthroscopy. Unfortunately, the reports of arthroscopy outcome are also open and uncontrolled clinical case descriptions with nonspecific criteria for success. For example, one report described over 4000 TMJs that were treated by arthroscopic surgery; only 9% of the surgical procedures was unsuccessful. The surgery was considered to have failed if open surgery was required after arthroscopic surgery.[35]

The success that has been reported for the use of arthroscopic surgery in the treatment of disk displacements without reduction does not mean that arthroscopy is a panacea for all disorders afflicting the TMJ. It also does not mean that every disk displacement without reduction benefits from the procedure. To achieve any long-term resolution, the etiologic factors must be identified during accurate preoperative treatment. There are numerous etiologic factors that can be identified; among these factors are clenching parafunctional habits, skeletal and occlusal dysplasias, environmental stress, and a history of trauma. A patient should not be considered a surgical candidate merely because appliance therapy and other treatments have failed. Some etiologic factors, such as nocturnal bruxism, have no current treatment; in patients with such conditions arthroscopic treatment is not successful. In patients with severe skeletal dysplasias requiring orthognathic surgery the arthroscopic procedure has traditionally been performed before any such surgery. Whether these patients should undergo TMJ surgery before, concurrent with, or after the orthognathic surgery is still debated.

SUMMARY

Well-designed and controlled research of the treatment of the human TMJ is needed. Preoperative evaluations should be performed (preferably at several points in time before the procedure) to ensure that spontaneous remission does not occur. Postoperative evaluations using the same measurements are also needed, and the methods of evaluation must be standardized, reproducible, and as objective as possible. These evaluations should be performed by experienced examiners who are unaware of a patient's status. The examiners should also evaluate patients who are not in the protocol so that the improvement of all patients is not expected. All patients entering the research protocol should meet a clear set of unambiguous criteria for inclusion and exclusion, and every entering patient should be tracked for the duration of the research project. Finally, the follow-up period must be long enough to provide an understanding of any tendency for relapse among the subjects. Until such data are available, the evidential basis for arthroscopy is subject to challenge.

REFERENCES

1. Moses, JJ; Sartoris, D; Glass, R, et al. The effect of arthroscopic surgical lysis and lavage of the superior joint space on TMJ disc position and mobility. J Oral Maxillofac Surg (1989), 47:674–678.
2. Ohnishi, M. Arthroscopy of the temporomandibular joint. Kokubyo Gakkai Zasshi (1975), 42:207–213.
3. Williams, RA; Laskin, DM. Arthroscopic examination of experi-mentally induced pathologic conditions of the rabbit temporomandibular joint. J Oral Surg (1980), 38:652–659.
4. Ohnishi, M. Clinical application of arthroscopy in the temporomandibular joint diseases. Bull Tokyo Med Dent Univ (1980), 27:141–150.
5. Hellsing, G; Holmlund, A; Nordenram, A; Wredmark, T. Arthroscopy of the temporomandibular joint: Examination of two patients with suspected disk derangement. Int J Oral Surg (1984), 13:69–74.
6. Murakami, K; Matsumoto, K; Lizzuka, T. Suppurative arthritis of the temporomandibular joint. Report of a case with special reference to arthroscopic observations. J Oral Maxillofac Surg (1984), 12:41.
7. Burke, RH. Temporomandibular joint diagnosis: Arthroscopy. J Craniomandib Pract (1985), 3:234–236.
8. Holmlund, A; Hellsing, G. Arthroscopy of the temporomandibular joint: An autopsy study. Int J Oral Surg (1985), 14:169.
9. Murakami, K; Matauki, M; Iizuka, T; Ono, T. Diagnostic arthroscopy of the TMJ: Differential diagnoses in patients with limited jaw opening. J Craniomandib Pract (1986), 4:118–126.
10. Goss, AN; Bosanquet, AG. Temporomandibular joint arthroscopy. J Oral Maxillofac Surg (1986), 44:614–617.
11. Eriksson, L; Westesson, P. Deterioration of temporary silicone implant in the temporomandibular joint: A clinical and arthroscopic follow-up study. Oral Surg Oral Med Oral Pathol (1986), 62:2.
12. Liedberg, J; Westesson, PL. Diagnostic accuracy of upper compartment arthroscopy of the temporomandibular joint: Correlation with postmortem morphology. Oral Surg Oral Med Oral Pathol (1986), 62:618–624.
13. Heffez, L; Blaustein, D. Diagnostic arthroscopy of the temporomandibular joint. Oral Surg Oral Med Oral Pathol (1987), 64:653–670.
14. Goss, AN; Bosanquet, AG; Tideman, H. The accuracy of temporomandibular joint arthroscopy. J Craniomaxillofac Surg (1987), 15:99–102.
15. Blaustein, D; Heffez, L. Diagnostic arthroscopy of the temporomandibular joint. Oral Surg Oral Med Oral Pathol (1988), 65:135–141.
16. Tarro, AW. Arthroscopic diagnosis and surgery of the temporomandibular joint. J Oral Maxillofac Surg (1988), 46:282–289.
17. McCain, JP. Arthroscopy of the human temporomandibular joint. J Oral Maxillofac Surg (1988), 46:648–655.
18. McCain, JP; de la Rua, H. Arthroscopic observation and treatment of synovial chondromatosis of the temporomandibular joint. Int J Oral Maxillofac Surg (1989), 18:233–236.
19. Bibb, CA; Pullinger, AG; Baldioceda, F; et al. Temporomandibular joint comparative imaging: Diagnostic efficacy of arthroscopy compared to tomography and arthrography. Oral Surg Oral Med Oral Pathol (1989), 68:352–359.
20. Sanders, B. Arthroscopic surgery of the temporomandibular joint: Treatment of internal derangement with persistent closed lock. Oral Surg Oral Med Oral Pathol (1986), 62:361–372.
21. Nuelle, DG; Alpern, MC; Ufema, JW. Arthroscopic surgery of the temporomandibular joint. Angle Orthod (1986), 56:118.
22. Nuelle, D; Alpern, M; Ufema, J. An arthroscopic perspective of the temporomandibular joint. J Craniomandib Pract (1987), 56:110.
23. Indresano, AT. Arthroscopic surgery of the temporomandibular joint: Report of 64 patients with long-term follow-up. J Oral Maxillofac Surg (1989), 47:439–441.
24. Israel, HA; Roser, SM. Patient response to temporomandibular joint arthroscopy: Preliminary findings in 24 patients. J Oral Maxillofac Surg (1989), 47:570–573.
25. Israel, HA. Technique for placement of a discal traction suture during temporomandibular joint arthroscopy. J Oral Maxillofac Surg (1989), 47:311–313.
26. Montgomery, MT; Van Sickels, JE; Harms SE; Thrash, WJ. Arthroscopic TMJ surgery: Effects on signs, symptoms, and disc position. J Oral Maxillofac Surg (1989), 47:1263–1271.
27. White, RD. Retrospective analysis of 100 consecutive surgical arthroscopies of the temporomandibular joint. J Oral Maxillofac Surg (1989), 47:1014–1021.

28. Gabler, MJ; Greene, CS; Palacios, E; Perry, HT. Effect of arthroscopic temporomandibular joint surgery on articular disk position. J Craniomandib Dis Fac Oral Pain (1989), 3:191–202.
29. Moses, JJ; Poker, ID. TMJ arthroscopic surgery: An analysis of 237 patients. J Oral Maxillofac Surg (1989), 47:790–794.
30. Ohnishi, M. Arthroscopic surgery for hypermobility and recurrent mandibular dislocation. Oral and Maxillofacial Surgery Clinics of North America (1989), 1:153.
31. Tarro, AW. Arthroscopic treatment of anterior disc displacement: A preliminary report. J Oral Maxillofac Surg (1989), 47:353–358.
32. Sanders, B; Kaminishi, R; Buoncristiani, R; Davis, C. Arthroscopic surgery for treatment of temporomandibular joint hypomobility after mandibular sagittal osteotomy. Oral Surg Oral Med Oral Pathol (1990), 69:539–541.
33. Forman, D; Jaffe, J. Facial pain treated by temporomandibular joint arthroscopy and styloidectomy: Report of case. J Am Dent Assoc (1990), 120:324.
34. Clark, GT; Moody, DG; Sanders, B. Arthroscopic treatment of temporomandibular joint locking resulting from disc derangement: Two-year results. J Oral Maxillofac Surg (1991), 49:157–164.
35. Tarro, AW. TMJ arthroscopic diagnosis and surgery: Clinical experience with 152 procedures over a 2½-year period. J Craniomandib Pract (1991), 9:107–119.
36. Forman, D. Success with temporomandibular joint arthroscopic surgery. Dent Clin North Am (1990), 34:135–141.
37. Holmlund, AB. Arthroscopy of the temporomandibular joint: Technique and indications. Ann Acad Med Singapore (1989), 18:541–547.
38. Baldioceda, F; Pullinger, A; Bibb, C. Distribution and histological character of condylar osseous defects. J Dent Res (1987), 66:319.
39. Pullinger, A; Baldioceda, F; Bibb, C. Prediction of TMJ articular surface configuration from condylar osseous outline. J Dent Res (1987), 66:338.
40. Hilsabeck, RB; Laskin, DM. Arthroscopy and the temporomandibular joint of the rabbit. J Oral Surg (1978), 36:938–943.
41. Kurita, K; Bronstein, SL; Westesson PL; Sternby, NH. Arthroscopic diagnosis of perforation and adhesions of the temporomandibular joint: Correlation with postmortem morphology. Oral Surg Oral Med Oral Pathol (1989), 68:130–134.
42. Eckerdal, O. Correlation between the tomographic image and the anatomy. Acta Radiol Suppl (Stockh) (1973), 329:52–73.
43. Hansson, T; Oberg, T. Arthrosis and deviation in form in the temporomandibular joint: A macroscopic study on a human autopsy material. Acta Odontol Scand (1977), 35:167–174.
44. Westesson, PL; Rohlin, M. Internal derangement related to osteoarthrosis in temporomandibular joint autopsy specimens. Oral Surg Oral Med Oral Pathol (1984), 57:17–21.
45. Solberg, WK; Hansson, TL; Nordstorm, B. The temporomandibular joint in young adults at autopsy: A morphologic classification and evaluation. J Oral Rehabil (1985), 12:303–321.
46. Hansson, T; Oberg, T; Carlsson, GE; Kopp, S. Thickness of the soft tissue layers and the articular disc in the temporomandibular joint. Acta Odontol Scand (1977), 35:77–83.
47. Holmlund, A; Hellsing, G; Wredmark, T. Arthroscopy of the temporomandibular joint. A clinical study. Int J Oral Maxillofac Surg (1986), 15:715–721.
48. Blackwood, HJJ. Arthritis of the mandibular joint. Br Dent J (1963), 115:317–326.
49. Moffett, BC; Johnson, LC; McCabe, JB; Askew, HC. Articular remodeling in the adult human temporomandibular joint. Am J Anat (1964), 115:119–142.
50. Sokoloff, L. The Biology of Degenerative Joint Disease. Chicago: The University of Chicago Press (1969).
51. Oberg, T; Carlsson, GE; Fajers, CM. The temporomandibular joint. A morphologic study on a human autopsy material. Acta Odontol Scand (1971), 29:349–384.
52. Akerman, S; Rohlin, M; Kopp, S. Bilateral degenerative changes and deviation in form of temporomandibular joints: An autopsy study of elderly individuals. Acta Odontol Scand (1984), 42:205–214.
53. Holmlund, A; Hellsing, G. Arthroscopy of the temporomandibular joint: Occurrence and location of osteoarthrosis and synovitis in a patient material. Int J Oral Maxillofac Surg (1988), 17:36–40.
54. Murakami, K; Hoshino, K. Regional anatomical nomenclature and arthroscopic terminology in human temporomandibular joints. Okajimas Folia Anat Jpn (1982), 58:745–760.
55. Murakami, K; Ito, K. Arthroscopy of the temporomandibular joint (2nd report): Arthroscopic anatomy and histologic studies of human cadavers. Arthroscopy (1982), 7:1.
56. Murakami, K; Hoshino, K. Histological studies on the inner surfaces of the articular cavities of human temporomandibular joints with special reference to arthroscopic observations. Anat Anz (1985), 160:167.
57. Bronstein, SL. Diagnostic and operative arthroscopy: Historical perspectives and indications. Oral Maxillofac Surg Clin N Am (1989), 1:59.
58. Murakami, K; Ono, T. Temporomandibular joint arthroscopy by inferolateral approach. Int J Oral Maxillofac Surg (1986), 15:410–417.
59. Riessner, D. Surgical procedure in tumors of parotid gland: Preservation of facial nerve and prevention of postoperative fistulas. AMA Arch Surg (1952), 65:831.
60. Furnas, DW. Landmarks for the trunk and the temporofacial division of the facial nerve. Br J Surg (1965), 52:694.
61. Pitanguy, I; Ramos, AS. The frontal branch of the facial nerve: The importance of its variations in face lifting. Plast Reconstr Surg (1966), 38:352.
62. Loeb, R. Technique for preservation of the temporal branches of the facial nerve during face-lift operations. Br J Plast Surg (1970), 23:390.
63. Baker, DC; Conley, J. Avoiding facial nerve injuries in rhytidectomy: Anatomical variations and pitfalls. Plast Reconstr Surg (1979), 64:781.
64. Al-Kayat, A; Bramley, P. A modified pre-auricular approach to the temporomandibular joint and malar arch. Br J Oral Surg (1979), 17:91.
65. Ozersky, D; Baek, SM; Biller, HF. Percutaneous identification of the temporal branch of the facial nerve. Ann Plast Surg (1980), 4:276.
66. Westesson, PL; Eriksson, L; Liedberg, J. The risk of damage to facial nerve, superficial temporal vessels, disk, and articular surfaces during arthroscopic examination of the temporomandibular joint. Oral Surg Oral Med Oral Pathol (1986), 62:124–127.
67. Sanders, B; Buoncristiani, R. Diagnostic and surgical arthroscopy of the temporomandibular joint: Clinical experience with 137 procedures over a 2-year period. J Craniomandib Dis Fac Oral Pain (1987), 1:202–213.
68. Moses, JJ; Poker, ID. Temporomandibular joint arthroscopy: The endaural approach. Int J Oral Maxillofac Surg (1989), 18:347–351.
69. Loughner, BA; Larkin, LH; Mahan, PE. Discomalleolar and anterior malleolar ligaments: Possible causes of middle ear damage during temporomandibular joint surgery. Oral Surg Oral Med Oral Pathol (1989), 68:14–22.
70. Herzog, S; Fiese, R. Persistent foramen of huschke: Possible risk factor for otologic complications after arthroscopy of the temporomandibular joint. Oral Surg Oral Med Oral Pathol (1989), 68:267–270.
71. Howerton, DW; Zysset, M. Anatomy of the temporomandibular joint and related structures with surgical anatomic considerations. Oral Maxillofac Surg Clin N Am (1989), 1:229.
72. Greene, MW; Hackney, FL; Van Sickels, JE. Arthroscopy of the temporomandibular joint: An anatomic perspective. J Oral Maxillofac Surg (1989), 47:386–389.
73. Pogrel, MA; Kaban, LB. The role of a temporalis fascia and muscle flap in temporomandibular joint surgery. J Oral Maxillofac Surg (1990), 48:14–19.
74. Murakami, K; Ito, K. Arthroscopy of the temporomandibular joint. In Watanabe, M, ed. Arthroscopy of Small Joints. Tokyo: Igaku-Shoin (1985), 128–139.
75. Ohnishi, M. (In Japanese) Kokubyo Gakkai Zasshi (1982), 31:487–512.
76. Ohnishi, M. Arthroscopy (1984), 9:43–48.
77. Ohnishi, M. Arthroscopic surgery of temporomandibular joint

diseases: No. 173. Abstract of a lecture presented at the Ninth ICOMS Conference, Vancouver, Canada, 1986.

78. Wilkes, CH. Arthroscopy of the temporomandibular joint in patients with the TMJ pain-dysfunction syndrome. Minn Med (1978), 61:645.

79. Clark, GT; Seligman, DA; Solberg, WK; Pullinger, AG. Guidelines for the examination and diagnosis of temporomandibular disorders. J Craniomandib Dis (1989), 3:7.

80. Piper, M; Chuong, R. Intraoperative assessment of discal position using C-arm arthrography during arthroscopic surgery (abstract). J Oral Maxillofac Surg (1987), 45:M3.

81. Braun, BL. The effect of physical therapy intervention on incisal opening after temporomandibular joint surgery. Oral Surg Oral Med Oral Pathol (1987), 64:544–548.

82. Van Sickels, JE; Nishioka, GJ; Hegewald, MD; Neal, GD. Middle ear injury resulting from temporomandibular joint arthroscopy. J Oral Maxillofac Surg (1987), 45:962–965.

83. Kondoh, T. Arthroscopic traction suture for clicking and hypermobility of the temporomandibular joint. Abstract of a lecture presented at the Seventy-second Annual Meeting and Scientific Sessions of the American Association of Oral and Maxillofacial Surgery, September 1990.

84. McCarty, WL; Farrar, WB. Surgery for internal derangements of the temporomandibular joint. J Prosthet Dent (1979), 42:191–196.

85. Brown, W. Internal derangement of the temporomandibular joint: Review of 241 patients following meniscectomy. Can J Surg (1980), 23:30.

86. American Association of Oral and Maxillofacial Surgery: Criteria for TMJ meniscus surgery. Chicago: American Association of Oral and Maxillofacial Surgery (1984).

87. Mercuri, LG; Campbell, RL; Shamaskin, RG. Intra-articular meniscus dysfunction surgery. Oral Surg (1982), 54:613.

88. Dolwick, MF. Surgical management. In: Helms, CA, Katzberg, RW, and Dolwick, MF, eds. Internal Derangements of the Temporomandibular Joint. San Francisco: Radiology Research and Education Foundation (1983).

89. Stith, HE. Surgical treatment of internal derangements of the temporomandibular joint: Review of 198 joints. Lecture presented at the American Association of Oral and Maxillofacial Surgery Annual Meeting, New York, New York, 1984.

90. Weinberg, S. Eminectomy and meniscoplasty for internal derangements of the temporomandibular joint. Oral Surg (1984), 57:241.

PART 3

Technology

Twelve

Temporomandibular Joint Arthroscopic Photography and Documentation Techniques

RALPH D. BUONCRISTIANI, D.D.S.

Since the late 1980s, arthroscopy has become recognized as an effective diagnostic and surgical therapeutic modality for internal derangements of the temporomandibular joint (TMJ). As a result, there has been an increase in the number of articles and books published on the subject. These publications often include photographs of arthroscopically observed joint pathology. High-quality intraarticular images are necessary for these publications.

Arthroscopic photography of the TMJ presents some unique difficulties not encountered in other types of arthroscopic photography owing to the small size of the scopes used. High-quality photographic representations of joint anatomy and pathology are needed for the advancement of this surgical technique.

HISTORICAL BACKGROUND

Like arthroscopy, arthroscopic photography is a highly equipment-dependent technique. Some of the significant innovations and refinements in endoscopic equipment, such as improved optics and light sources, allowed its use with photography and later with video recording equipment. A few of these developments merit mention.

The first documented endoscopic instrument was described in 1806 by Phillip Bozzini.[5] This instrument was not given practical recognition until 1853, when Desormeaux developed a urethroscope. All of these early instruments employed illumination from a burning candle or a lamp. The adaptation of an electrically heated platinum loop positioned at the end of the instrument, first proposed in 1857 by the dentist Julius Brucke, increased the effective illumination. Max Nitze adapted and incorporated this concept along with an image-conducting lens system into early endoscopes.[2,6]

In 1894, Nitze developed the first successful photographic endoscope. Using a rotating glass disk and a prism system adapted to a cystoscope, the image could be directed either to the eyepiece or to a photographic emulsion on the disk.[2] The disk could be rotated as well, allowing multiple images to be recorded. Edison's invention of the electric light bulb in 1880 led to the replacement of the electrically heated platinum loop on the end of the endoscope, thereby improving the reliability of the instrument and increasing the quantity of light. Although not used on Nitze's original photographic cystoscope, the electric light bulb positioned at the end of the scope was later adapted to endoscopic photography.

The first arthroscopic photographs, both still and 16mm motion-picture images, were taken by Kenji Takagi in 1932.[2]

CURRENT PHOTOGRAPHIC TECHNOLOGY

High-quality arthroscopic photographs and images can be obtained using various techniques. Video tape recording has been available for several years and provides a convenient and accurate motion picture record of diagnostic and surgical procedures. In the past, static image production for publication has primarily been performed using 35mm cameras. With the expansion of video electronics technology, video printers and video floppy disk recorders have become good alternatives for simple, quality image production. This chapter discusses static images only. The topic of motion picture video tape recording is beyond the scope of this chapter.

Camera photography is the most readily available means of producing static images and is the most commonly used technique to produce images for publication. This method yields the best quality picture of all image production techniques (Fig. 12–1). Some relatively sophisticated camera equipment is needed to

photograph directly through the arthroscope. The basic setup requires a 35mm single-lens reflex camera with a lens of 100mm or greater. Most high-quality 35mm cameras can be adapted for this use. A coupler to attach the camera lens to the arthroscope is also needed. Some additional features are desirable; these include a spot-metering system for exposure calibration, a power winder, a magnification lens system built into the camera coupler, a data-back camera attachment for photograph identification, and highly light-sensitive film.

The light-metering systems on standard 35mm cameras are designed to evaluate the available light and adjust the film exposure accordingly. Different cameras perform this exposure evaluation, or metering, in different ways. The area metered may be the entire viewfinder field or only selected areas of this field.

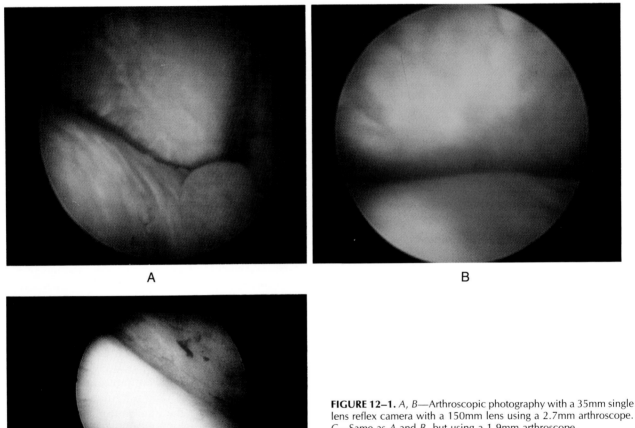

A

B

C

FIGURE 12–1. *A, B*—Arthroscopic photography with a 35mm single lens reflex camera with a 150mm lens using a 2.7mm arthroscope. *C*—Same as *A* and *B*, but using a 1.9mm arthroscope.

Thirty-five–millimeter cameras commonly use a system for center weighting or averaging the light intensity within the entire viewfinder.

In arthroscopic photography, the image created by the arthroscope is limited to the center of the camera's viewfinder screen. The image consists of a disk surrounded by a black background. The image does not cover the entire light-sensitive screen. If the camera were to obtain exposure information from this black background area outside of the image, the camera's metering system would attempt to compensate for it. This may result in an overexposed image, with the black background area appearing gray and the disk (the actual image area) appearing too bright on the final photograph. A metering system for arthroscopic photography should ignore this black area and should obtain all of its exposure information from a spot at the center only; hence, the need for a spot-metering system. If this is not available, exposure compensation can be accomplished manually by intentionally underexposing the film. Some experimentation is required to determine the correct settings.

The size of the image is determined by the lens system. The smaller the focal length, the smaller the image on the slide. Ideally, the slide frame should be filled by the image. The literature on arthroscopic photography suggests that the minimum magnification needed to obtain an adequately sized image is achieved using a 100mm lens.[3,7] Arthroscopy of the TMJ uses very small diameter arthroscopes that produce correspondingly small images. For TMJ arthroscopic photography lenses of 150–200mm are recommended for adequate magnification of the image (Fig. 12–2).

There is a tradeoff between image magnification and exposure time. As the image is enlarged, the available light is decreased because it is spread over a larger area. Longer exposure times are therefore necessary in TMJ arthroscopic photography. This necessitates high-speed (very light-sensitive) film. Film speeds of ASA 400 or greater are recommended. Kodak's Ektachrome 400 has proved to be a good film for producing slide photographs.[3]

A camera adaptor suitable to connect the arthroscope to the camera is required. This adaptor includes both a threaded ring with which to screw it onto the end of the camera-lens system and a fitting to go over the ocular end of the arthroscope. This adaptor may contain a magnification lens that additionally enlarges the image (Fig. 12–3).

The light sources used for arthroscopy are generally adequate for most arthroscopic photography. Some light sources have an auto-sensing capability to adjust illumination. As the light sources are coupled to the video camera to provide feedback and automatic adjustment of the light level, it is important to turn off any auto-sensing function. Feedback from the video camera is not available when a photographic camera is being used. Light intensity should be adjusted manually to ensure comfortable viewing.

Cameras and arthroscope lens systems both have an optical point of reference at which the image is focused at its brightest point. This is referred to as the *exit pupil*. In a camera this is usually located behind the front-lens element in the general location of the iris diaphragm that determines the aperture setting (f-stop) in routine photography (Fig. 12–4). When photographs are taken through the arthroscope, the position of the exit pupil in the camera-lens system is determined by the lens system in the arthroscope. It is therefore best to leave the camera-lens aperture (f-stop) wide open.[1]

The actual aperture setting is controlled by the size of the ocular lens of the arthroscope. The f-stop is calculated by dividing the lens focal length by the size of the aperture. For example, a scope with a 2-mm ocular lens using a 150mm camera lens results in an f-stop of 75 ($150/2 = 75$).[2] A benefit of these very small aperture settings is an increase in the relative depth of the field. This ensures that more of the image is in focus. Most images will be in good focus if the camera lens is adjusted to a focal distance of 2–3 feet.

DISADVANTAGES OF PHOTOGRAPHY THROUGH AN ARTHROSCOPE

One of the major disadvantages of camera photography is that bringing a camera into the surgical field breaks sterility. A second disadvantage is that a camera can be clumsy and unwieldy. The difference in the relative weight of a camera versus that of a scope can result in instrument breakage. A camera's size and weight difference also present difficulties in positioning. Finally, the time involved to change to the photographic camera from the video camera prolongs the operating time significantly.

PHOTOGRAPHY FROM THE VIDEO MONITOR

The surgeon who does not have the specialized attachments and equipment needed for direct intraarticular photography through an arthroscope can obtain good quality images directly from video tape recordings viewed on a high-quality television monitor. However, several points must be taken into account if satisfactory images are to be produced. Any camera with adjustments for focus and exposure is satisfactory for this

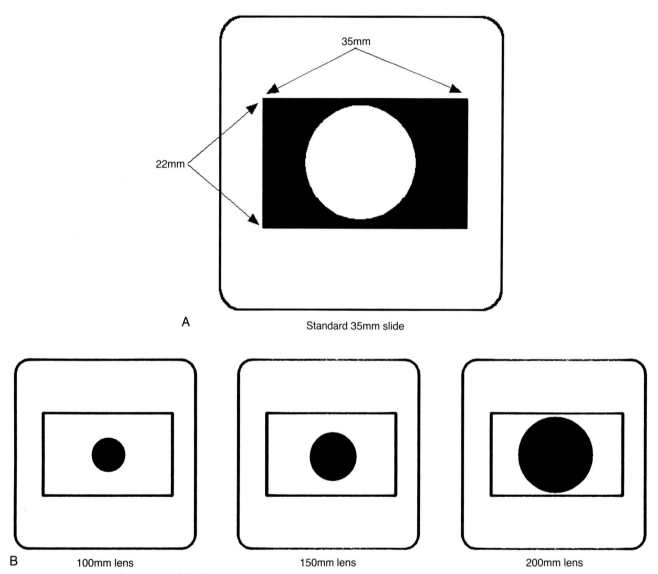

FIGURE 12–2. *A*—Standard 35mm slide demonstrating areas of ideal image size and placement. *B*—Standard 35mm slides demonstrating various image sizes with varying lens systems.

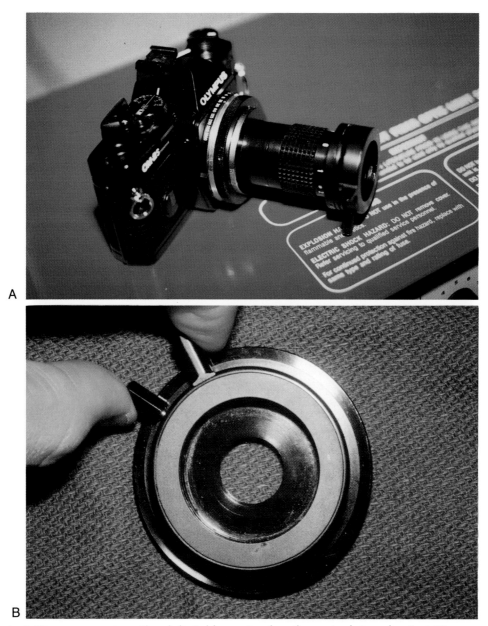

FIGURE 12–3. *A*—A 35mm camera setup with a dedicated lens system for arthroscopic photography. *B*—A 35mm camera lens adaptor to couple a standard lens to the ocular lens of the arthroscope.

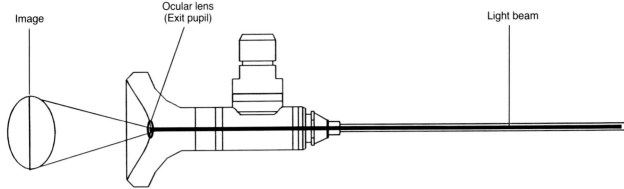

Image
Ocular lens (Exit pupil)
Light beam

FIGURE 12–4. Light path through the arthroscope. The exit pupil determines the lens aperture (f-stop).

purpose. The exposure of the film can be gauged using the exposure meter on the camera. The f-stop should be set to obtain a properly exposed image, but narrow or wide aperture settings generally do not alter the image quality. However, it is important to set the exposure time. The exposure time should be 1/30 second or longer (preferably 1/15 or 1/8 second). Exposure times less than 1/30 second (i.e., 1/60 or shorter) result in the appearance of dark streaks across the image. This is a result of how the television creates the image we see.

The image on the monitor screen comprises a series of horizontal lines drawn across the screen by a moving electron beam. These lines are drawn across the screen sequentially from top to bottom, reproducing each full image 30 times/second.[4] It is the succession of each of these individual images recorded on the videotape that gives the appearance of motion on the video monitor, just as the succession of still images on a movie film gives the illusion of motion. If the camera exposure is set for less than 1/30 second the image will be incompletely drawn. This will result in the appearance of a dark streak or band across the photograph (Fig. 12–5).

Direct offscreen photography should be performed in a darkened room in order to avoid the glare from the monitor screen. Flash equipment is of no benefit and actually detracts from or spoils the images. A portion of the videotape where the image is still should be used because this ensures less distortion when more than one image is drawn on the monitor during the exposure of the photograph (Fig. 12–6A).

The advantages of creating images using direct off-screen photography include the relative ease of production and the need for only relatively simple equipment. There are, however, several disadvantages. For example, the quality of an image is dependent on the quality of the television monitor. Furthermore, color balance and quality are only as good as that which the monitor is able to produce. The resolution of the final image is also limited by the resolution of the monitor as the detail of the final image is dependent on the number of horizontal scan lines drawn. Standard television monitors have approximately 250 horizontal lines of resolution, and standard video tape recorders record only about 280 lines of resolution. A low-resolution monitor may result in the appearance of horizontal scan lines on the final image.

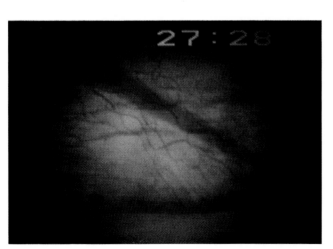

FIGURE 12–5. Photograph demonstrating a dark streak through the image due to short exposure time when photographing directly off the video monitor.

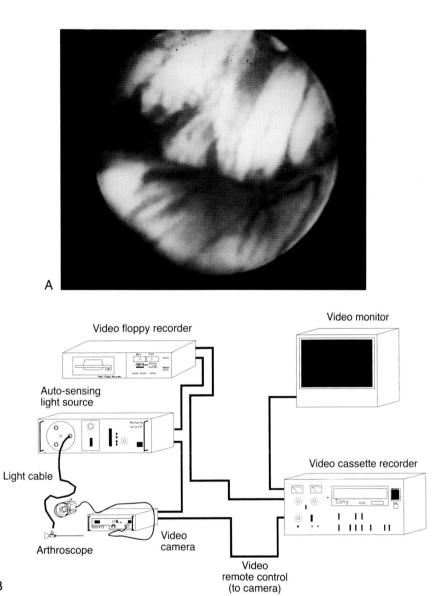

FIGURE 12–6. *A*—Arthroscopic view of the temporomandibular joint as photographed off the video monitor. Note the coarse lines of horizontal resolution. *B*—Electronic hookups including video recording equipment for both still and motion picture images.

VIDEO IMAGE RECORDING

It is possible to produce high-quality video photographic images. The electronic signal produced by the video camera for the monitor can be directed to other electronic equipment for processing into photographs or prints. This is advantageous as it does not require additional equipment in the surgical field as does camera photography. The equipment is merely connected to the current video signal (Fig. 12–6*B*). A still image can be processed by a thermal printer attached to the video source or can be recorded on video floppy disk for later retrieval and processing.

Video printers have been available for several years. Unfortunately, those available offer poor color and contrast reproduction. Newer units are able to produce images that approach photographic quality. Images can also be produced using a Polaroid film recorder. This device can produce high-resolution 35mm or instant-print–type photos from a video source.

Individual images can also be recorded on a video floppy disk recorder for later processing (Fig. 12–7). This device records the video signal in analog format on a small floppy disk similar to those used on computers (Fig. 12–8). Up to 50 images can be recorded for later viewing. The individual images can be reviewed and only the best selected and produced as photographs or thermal prints (Fig. 12–9). Video floppy recorders are also less expensive than thermal printers or film recorders.

A key factor limiting the quality of a video image is the horizontal resolution of the monitor. As with direct photography using a television monitor, the number of horizontal scan lines that make up the picture determines the detail of the final photographs. Most video cameras in common use have horizontal resolutions of 280–300 lines. Newer super VHS cameras have resolutions of 360 lines, and cameras may be capable of resolutions of 430 lines within the near future. Video tape recorders are able to record 280 lines of resolution, and video floppy disk recorders can record 380 lines of resolution.

As video technology improves, the resolution of video images approaches that of photographs. The ease of use of video imaging allows surgeons who are less skilled in the art of photography to produce publication-quality images. The convenience of video imaging also makes it possible to obtain a greater number of photographs without unduly prolonging operating time.

PHOTOGRAPHIC RECONSTRUCTION OF THE JOINT

Sequential images of the entire TMJ superior joint space can be created and then assembled to obtain a complete view of the whole joint. Such a representation would be exceedingly difficult to create using a camera. Using the video floppy disk recorder, individual images can be rapidly recorded in sequence and then later assembled and printed in photograph form (Fig. 12–10). In order to illustrate a specific surgical procedure, sequential images can be recorded, printed, and presented in chronologic order.

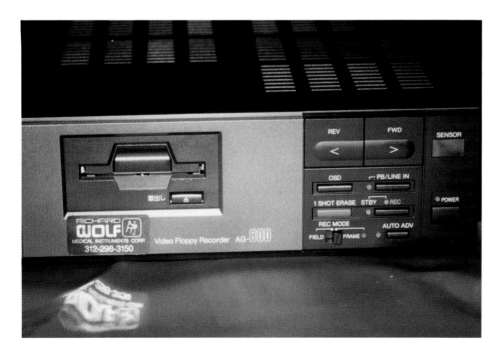

FIGURE 12–7. Video floppy recorder for the recording of still video images.

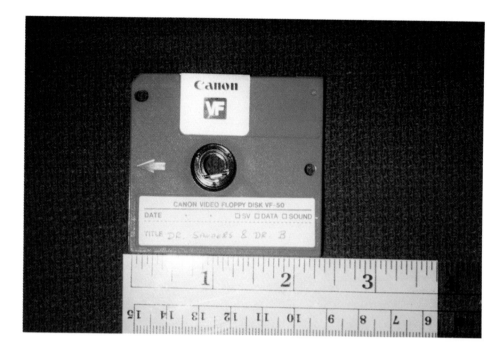

FIGURE 12–8. Video floppy disk for use in the video floppy recorder. The disk can hold up to 50 images for later processing into photographic images or video prints.

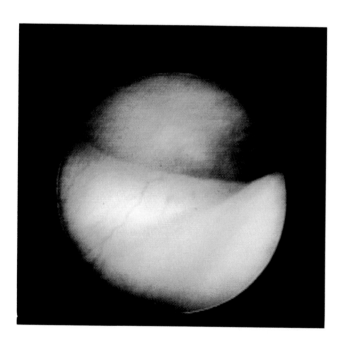

FIGURE 12–9. A processed image recorded on a video floppy disk. Note the much higher quality of the image due to the finer (more numerous) lines of horizontal resolution.

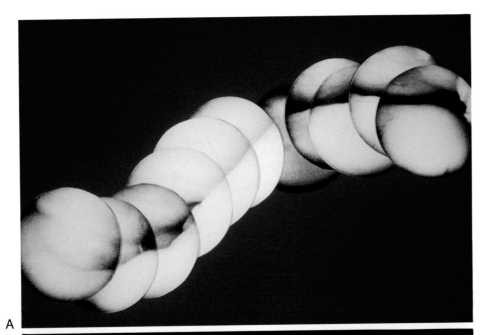

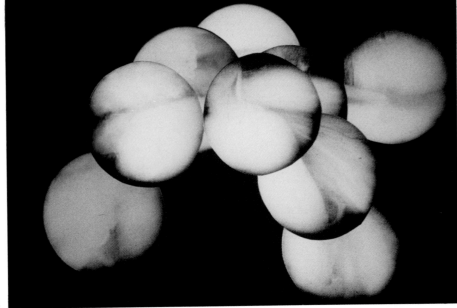

FIGURE 12–10. *A*—View of a right temporomandibular joint superior compartment reconstructed with a series of still images recorded on the video floppy recorder. *B*—Reconstructed view of a right temporomandibular joint with a large central perforation showing the head of the condyle.

REFERENCES

1. McGinty, J. Photography in arthroscopy. *In*: Casscelles, SW, ed. Arthroscopy: Diagnostic and Surgical Practice. Philadelphia: Lea & Febiger (1984), 9–15.
2. Medicine and early photography. Ciba Found Symp (1942), 4:1345–1355.
3. Dandy, DJ. Photography and television. *In*: Dandy, DJ. Arthroscopic Management of the Knee. London: Churchill Livingstone (1987), 28–35.

4. Pennington, D of the Richard Wolf Medical Instrument Corporation. Personal communication, 1986.
5. Wetterman, LA. From endoscopy to arthroscopy. *In*: O'Connor, RL. Arthroscopy. Philadelphia: JB Lippincott Co. (1977), 1–13.
6. Watanabe, M; Bechtol, R; Nottage, W. History of arthroscopic surgery. *In*: Sharriaree, HL, ed. O'Connor's Textbook of Arthroscopic Surgery. Philadelphia: JB Lippincott Co. (1984), 1–6.
7. Sharriaree, HL. Recording arthroscopic procedures. *In*: Sharriaree, HL, ed. O'Connor's Textbook of Arthroscopic Surgery. Philadelphia: JB Lippincott Co. (1984), 37–41.

Thirteen

Arthroscopic Laser Surgery and Suturing for Temporomandibular Joint Disorders

MASATOSHI OHNISHI, D.D.S., Ph.D.

The temporomandibular joint (TMJ) is functionally complex and anatomically delicate. For this reason, a small lesion in the TMJ cavity can have severe functional consequences. Conventional open surgery has been used to treat small intraarticular lesions. This requires extensive surgical invasion and involves areas of tissue beyond the lesion itself. In order to reduce the number of postoperative complications we have employed arthroscopic methods, which are less invasive than conventional types of surgery, in the treatment of lesions confined to the TMJ cavity. We have developed a new method for dealing with TMJ lesions that utilizes a Nd:YAG (neodymium-yttrium-aluminum-garnet) laser and arthroscopic suturing.[1-8]

PRINCIPLE OF THE PROCEDURE

Since relaxation of the soft tissue structure of the TMJ and articular capsule is considered to be a cause of hypermobility, habitual dislocation, and disk displacement, conventional surgery for entering the joint and condensing it by suturing is performed at a site posterior to the disk. Arthroscopic surgery is performed to scar the synovial membrane of the posterior wall, especially at the site of the oblique protuberance. Subsequent inhibition of forward motion of the mandibular condyle and disk is caused by second-stage healing and contracture of the scar.[9,10] To achieve a more permanent outcome, the posterior margin of the disk is arthroscopically sutured at the posterior wall to inhibit forward shifting.

EXAMINATION BEFORE SURGERY

Arthroscopy is especially helpful in diagnosis as it enables the surgeon to directly observe the condition of the intraarticular wall. However, it is necessary to envision the overall condition of the joint. To this end the use of double-contrast arthrotomography or magnetic resonance imaging (MRI) is effective for observing relationships among the joint space, disk, synovial membrane, and condyle. We have developed a technique utilizing double-contrast computed tomography (CT) of the TMJ that enables the surgeon to conduct a detailed study of the condition of the mandibular condyle, the bone structure, the joint space, and the soft tissues of the disk and synovial membrane. The use of double-contrast CT of the TMJ is an important step in determining if arthroscopic surgery is indicated.[11]

SPECIAL ARTHROSCOPIC SURGICAL EQUIPMENT AND INSTRUMENTS FOR LASER SURGERY AND SUTURING

TMJ arthroscopy and arthroscopic surgery require the use of a system with a needle scope of the smallest

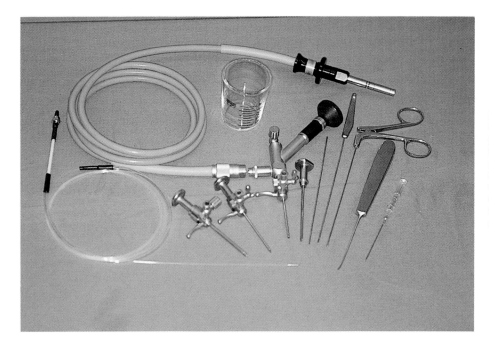

FIGURE 13–1. Instruments used in temporomandibular arthroscopic surgery: (from *left* to *right*) quartz fiber for neodymium-yttrium-aluminum-garnet (Nd:YAG) laser, guiding light, trocar (needle and double and single channel cannulas), surgical arthroscope, guiding needle, scalpel, forceps, suture needle, and lock-up needle.

possible diameter. For our work[12] we used Nd:YAG laser equipment (MYL-2 [Olympus Optical Co., Japan], Medilas 2, and 4ON6ON [MBB, Germany]). Quartz fibers 1.0 mm in diameter (Olympus Optic, SLT, MBB) were used for the guiding light (Figs. 13–1 and 13–2). Arthroscopic laser surgery was performed in the presence of intraarticular saline perfusion (30 ml/min), with a laser output of 20–35 watts and a perfusion temperature of less than 40°C.

A newly devised arthroscopic suture needle made of stainless steel was utilized in the procedure. It consists of two parts (a needle and its holder); its full length is 21 cm, approximately one half being the needle itself. The eye at the tip of the needle is 1.0 mm in diameter.

Depending on the operative case, either one-half–circle or one-third–circle needle tips were used (Fig. 13–3; see also Fig. 13–1). The suture material was 3–0 monofilament nylon.

ARTHROSCOPIC TECHNIQUE FOR LASER SURGERY AND SUTURING

The basic surgical procedures for arthroscopic laser surgery and arthroscopic suturing followed our usual method.[9] The entire procedure was carried out using a newly designed needle while the joint cavity was

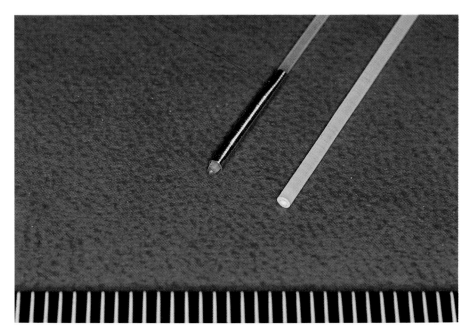

FIGURE 13–2. Laser quartz fibers (*left:* multiform fiber manufactured by MBB Co.; *right:* bare fiber manufactured by SLT Co.).

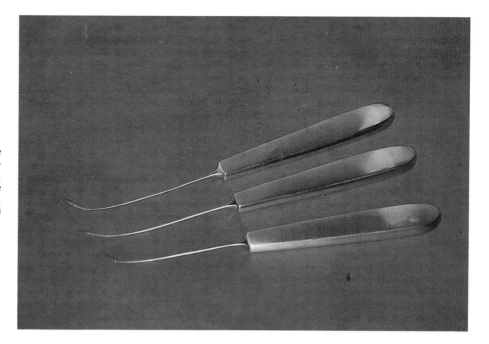

FIGURE 13–3. Arthroscopic suture needle with an eye 1.0 mm in diameter at its tip. Depending on the case, either 1/2-circle or 1/3-circleal needle tips are used. (Olympus Optical Co., Japan O. Leibinger GmBH, Germany)

viewed via either the double-channel cannula or the triangulation technique (Fig. 13–4).

Arthroscopy requires either that (1) two cannulas be inserted into the joint cavity (the triangulation technique), or that (2) a double-channel cannula (sheath) method using a newly developed needle-like rigid arthroscope (Olympus Optical Co., Japan) be employed.[13] In practice, a one-channel arthroscopic cannula is introduced into the upper joint cavity via the outer posterior puncture. Following observation of the joint interior, arthroscopic surgery is performed. In the first method, a one-channel cannula is introduced anteriorly into the upper joint cavity in the anterior part of the eminence. In the second method, a double-channel cannula (with an outer diameter of 3.8 mm × 2.0 mm) is introduced via a guide needle to replace the one-channel cannula already in place. Such manipulation allows both the arthroscope and the surgical instrument to be concurrently placed into the joint by either the first or the second method (Fig. 13–4). An Nd:YAG laser fiber probe is then inserted parallel to the optic tube of the arthroscope into the joint cavity through either the opening of the double-channel cannula or one of the cannulas if the triangulation technique is used (Figs. 13–5 and 13–6; see also Fig. 13–4).

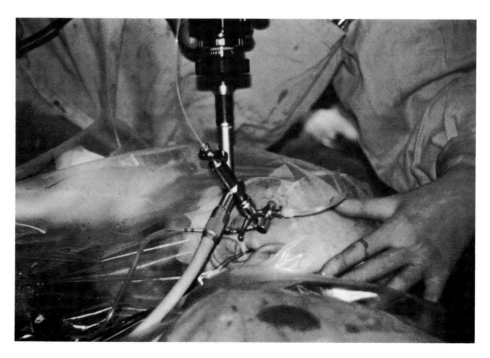

FIGURE 13–4. Arthroscopic laser surgery by the double-channel cannula method using a surgical arthroscope. A laser-guiding optical quartz fiber is inserted through a cannula lumen for the surgical instrument, and surgery is then performed with the aid of television monitoring.

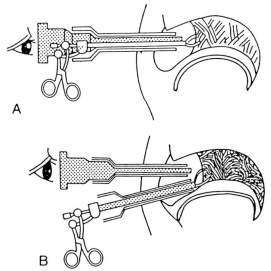

FIGURE 13–5. Arthroscopic surgical technique. *A*—Double-channel cannula method: An arthroscope and a surgical instrument are inserted simultaneously into the cannula and surgery is performed under visualization of the joint cavity. *B*—Triangulation technique.

ARTHROSCOPIC SURGICAL PROCEDURES

In patients with fibrous adhesions, laser cauterization and vaporization are performed to remove tissue fragments of the ruptured and torn synovial membrane and inner wall cartilage that result from the injury to the joint.

In patients with hypermobility (subluxation), habitual dislocation, anterior disk displacement, or any combination of these conditions, laser cauterization and vaporization was directed at the oblique protuberance in the upper joint cavity.[10] The aim is to produce coagulation in deep tissue and form a fresh wound on the surface of the synovial membrane behind the disk. Next, the disk was moved posteriorly and sutured to form an adhesion and a cicatrix between the posterior wall and the posterior aspect of the disk. The disk was moved backward by manipulation with an arthroscopic probe or a hook inserted into the joint cavity via an endaural puncture.[9] It is difficult to move the disk backward in patients with severe disk displacement without reduction. To assure adhesion of the posterior wall and the posterior disk tissue in these patients, the posterior tissue of the disk is sutured to the posterior wall of the joint and to the anterior wall of the external auditory canal by means of our arthroscopic suture method.[9,12]

The arthroscopic suture needle (see Fig. 13–3) is introduced at a position 10–15 mm anteroinferior to the eminence of the TMJ so that the curve of the needle tip advances from the anterior wall of the superior joint cavity into the cavity itself (Figs. 13–7 and 13–8; see also Fig. 13–6B). When the tip of the arthroscopic needle can be seen in the superior joint

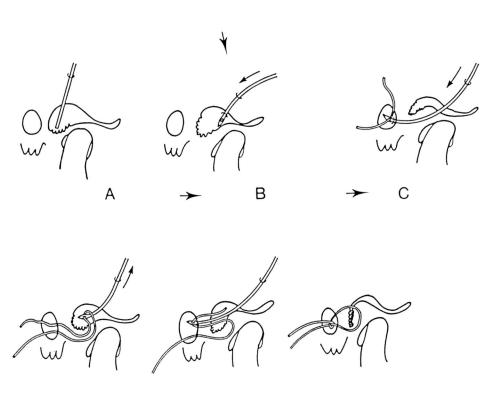

FIGURE 13–6. Schematic drawing of arthroscopic suturing technique. *A*—Burning (using a laser) or incision on the synovial surface to produce a fresh wound. *B*—Insertion of suture needle into the joint cavity. *C*—Puncture of the needle into the disk and its movement out of the external auditory meatus. The thread is passed through the hole of the needle. *D*—Movement of the needle back again into the joint cavity. *E*—Puncture of the needle again into the posterior wall and its movement out of the meatus. *F*—Tying of the thread.

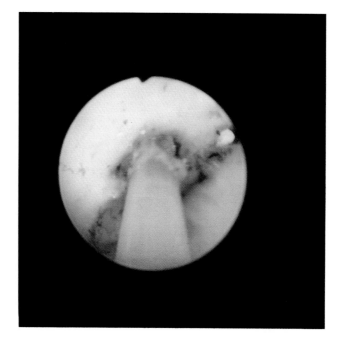

FIGURE 13–7. Arthroscopic finding during arthroscopic laser surgery. The tip of the laser probe is visible in the center.

cavity via the endoscopic TV camera, we carefully advance the needle tip and insert it into the edges of the fresh wound created at the posterior edge of the disk. The tip then is advanced until the needle's eye is exposed in the external auditory canal (Fig. 13–9; see also Fig. 13–6C). A suture is then threaded through the eye. The tip is again brought back into the joint cavity where the arthroscope is then manipulated (see Figs. 13–6D and 13–8). Next, the tip is inserted into the posterior wall tissue along the posterior edge of the fresh contralateral wound. As this is done, the

needle advances through the anteromural skin of the external auditory canal until the eye is exposed (see Fig. 13–6E).

When the suture is removed from the eye of the needle and is tied in the external auditory canal, the posterior edge of the articular disk and the posterior wall are approximated (see Fig. 13–6F).

If necessary, similar manipulations can be repeated while the suture needle is kept in the joint, thereby creating a continuous suture. To tie stitches, gauze can be used as a cushion to minimize damage to the

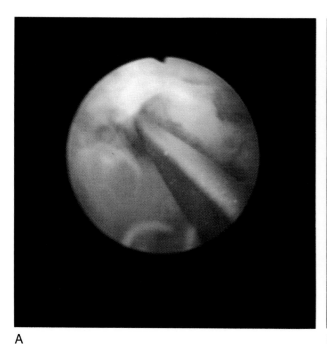

A

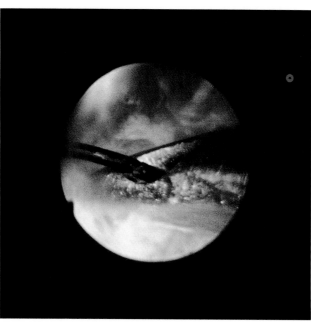

B

FIGURE 13–8. Arthroscopic findings during arthroscopic suturing in the stages depicted in Figures 13–6B (A) and 13–6D (B).

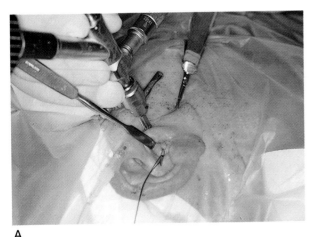

A

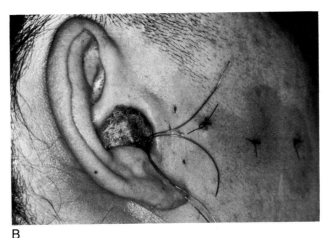

B

FIGURE 13–9. Findings during and after arthroscopic suturing. *A*—The needle tip is advanced until the needle's eye is exposed in the external auditory canal. *B*—When stitches are tied, gauze can be used as a cushion.

anteromural skin of the external auditory canal (see Fig. 13–9).

CLINICAL RESULTS

Eighty patients with varying disorders in 138 TMJs were selected from among those patients who visited our outpatient clinic from June 1986 to February 1990. These patients were diagnosed at clinical examinations as having intraarticular lesions that could benefit from arthroscopic laser surgery and arthroscopic suturing.

Seventeen of the 80 patients had fibrous adhesions (28 joints), 9 had fresh traumatic injuries (14 joints), 15 displayed hypermobility in the form of subluxation (26 joints), 15 experienced habitual dislocation (27 joints), and 24 had anterior disk displacement (37 joints).

Preoperatively the patients were evaluated based on a physical examination, arthrotomography, and double-contrast CT scanning of the TMJ.[9,11] Only those patients who failed to respond to more than 3 months of conservative therapy and who were suspected of having intraarticular mechanical symptoms were candidates for surgery.

Of the 17 patients who underwent the separation of fibrous adhesions of the TMJ to expand the range of mouth opening, 14 could open their mouths more than 35 mm after surgery. All 9 of the patients with acute traumatic injuries of the joint had mouth openings greater than 35 mm. Thirty patients with hypermobility were treated with an Nd:YAG laser to reduce the range of motion to within normal limits. Fifteen patients were judged to have subluxation, 13 of whom had successful surgical outcomes. The remaining 15 patients with habitual dislocations were all relieved of their symptoms.

There were 24 patients diagnosed with closed-lock.

They were treated with a combination of laser resection and arthroscopic suturing. The symptoms disappeared in 23 of the 24 patients following surgery.

Patients with fibrous adhesions of the TMJ began vigorous mandibular opening exercises shortly after surgery to prevent the recurrence of adhesions and to increase the range of mouth opening. Patients with subluxation, habitual dislocation, or disk displacements were required to restrict jaw movement after surgery to allow for adhesion of the posterior wall and the posterior disk. Jaw stabilization was achieved via loose intermaxillary fixation with gum rings for a 2–3-week period.

Overall, 92% of the 80 patients treated with combinations of arthroscopic laser and suture techniques were relieved of their symptoms.

Case Reports

Fibrous Adhesion. A 45-year-old female presented with an adhesion of the lateral wall of the left upper joint cavity. The patient subsequently underwent arthroscopic laser surgery. Joint cavity stenosis increased 5 months after surgery. However, the range of mouth opening increased from 17 mm before surgery to 38 mm after surgery.

Habitual Dislocation. A 69-year-old male presented with bilateral dislocation. Comparison of double-contrast CT scans performed before and 2 months after surgery indicated that the posterior disk tissue had thickened after surgery and was accompanied by a reduction in the forward shift tissue as well as of the disk. This patient underwent subsequent arthroscopic suturing (Fig. 13–10).

Anterior Disk Displacement. A 20-year-old female presented with bilateral disk displacement. Arthroscopic findings 5 months after surgery indicated cicatrix

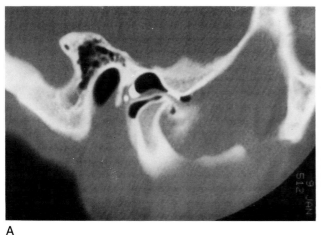
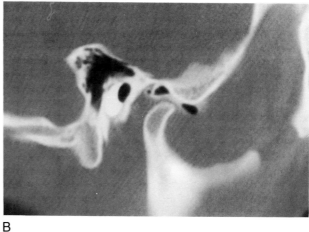

A   B

FIGURE 13–10. Habitual dislocation case: T.T., 69-year-old man, upper cavity of the right temporomandibular joint, double-contrast computed tomography (CT) scan, direct sagittal section. A—Dilatation of the joint cavity and marked relaxation of the inner wall are observed before surgery. B—The distance between the posterior disk and the posterior wall was abridged following surgery.

formation and a lack of elasticity in the posterior wall, the posterior disk tissue, and the oblique protuberance. In addition, the distance between the disk and the posterior wall during maximum mouth opening was abridged. A double-contrast CT scan supported the arthroscopic findings and also indicated a backward shift of the disk (Fig. 13–11).

DISCUSSION OF ARTHROSCOPIC LASER SURGERY

Although arthroscopic surgery is popular in the field of orthopedic surgery,[14,15] the use of lasers in arthroscopic surgery has been attempted primarily in Japan and in the United States.[16–18] If utilized properly, carbon dioxide, Nd:YAG, and argon lasers can all be used in arthroscopic surgery. Carbon dioxide lasers are

particularly appropriate for knee surgery, which involves the separation and the removal of torn tissue.

However, the lack of appropriate guidance for the intraarticular insertion of the carbon dioxide laser remains a problem. In 1980, Inoue studied the separation and the vaporization of synovial membranes, the meniscus, and the articular cartilage using a carbon dioxide laser.[18] He subsequently developed a carbon dioxide laser fiber with an outer diameter of 6.0 mm as well as an arthroscope for surgical use, and reported on the actual clinical application of these instruments. According to Inoue[18] the carbon dioxide laser is suitable for cauterizing the synovial membrane when set at a relatively high energy level. Conversely, the Nd:YAG laser is capable of causing heat injury to the synovial membrane when set at a relatively low energy level. Nd:YAG laser is particularly suited for surgery of the TMJ for the following reasons: (1) a guiding

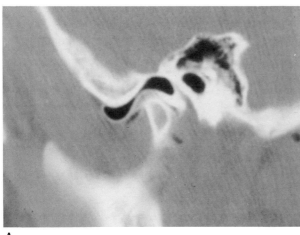
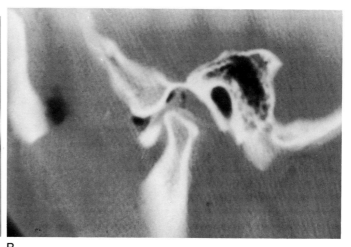

A   B

FIGURE 13–11. Anterior disc displacement case: M.T., 20-year-old female, upper cavity of the right temporomandibular joint, double-contrast CT scan, direct sagittal section. The positions of the mandibular head and disk are clearly different before (A) and after (B) surgery as viewed during maximum mouth opening. After the operation, abridgment of the distance between the posterior wall and the posterior disk was accompanied by a change in surface appearance. These findings are consistent with the arthroscopic findings.

optic fiber 0.5 or 1.0 mm in outer diameter is available and allows the laser to be easily inserted into the joint cavity; (2) the energy of the Nd:YAG laser is sufficient to reach a depth of 0.8–4.2 mm from the surface;[18,19] and (3) the Nd:YAG laser is a contact laser and is efficient for joint surgery. Besides being capable of resecting adhesions, the laser can produce extensive cicatrix formation in disorders where the aim of surgery is the reduction of joint mobility,[9,12,19] such as subluxation, habitual dislocation, and disk displacement.

ARTHROSCOPIC LASER SURGERY OF THE TMJ

Although we have been performing arthroscopic laser surgery for TMJ disorders since 1985,[19] we know of no other reports describing the use of this technique in joints as small as the TMJ. As it is difficult to perform complex surgical procedures with a laser in the narrow TMJ cavity, we have found that relying on touch is safer and more accurate in the use of laser radiation. For this reason, we use a direct-contact–type quartz fiber. Arthroscopic laser surgery is still of limited use and is confined to simple operations such as the incision, separation, and detachment of small areas of soft tissues (e.g., the synovial membrane, disk tissue, and cartilage). We perform laser surgery with our newly developed double-channel cannula method using a surgical arthroscope.[19] The primary objectives of Nd:YAG laser surgery are to coagulate, vaporize, and cauterize tissue in the TMJ cavity in order to separate fibrous adhesions and to form a fresh wound on the surface of the synovial membrane. Compared with the forceps and scalpel used for conventional surgery, the laser has a number of advantages. For example, it achieves the same results as other instruments without the use of mechanical force. Also, its energy output can be easily controlled. Good visualization of the joint cavity during surgery is also possible as the irrigation distends the joint and controls bleeding. Laser heat can be effectively controlled with the use of an irrigating solution (physiologic saline). Finally, by changing energy output, the laser radiation can have different effects on tissue and therefore can be used reliably to treat deep tissue as well as is achieved with surface laser radiation.[18,19]

ARTHROSCOPIC SUTURING TECHNIQUE IN THE TMJ

In 1989, we described procedures combining arthroscopy and suturing.[9] Such procedures were also described by Israel[20] and Tarro[21] that same year. In their work Israel and Tarro used arthroscopic suturing techniques for posterior distraction and immobilization in patients with anterior disk displacement. In contrast, our technique is used to achieve articular mobility control, to restrict the range of opening in cases of dislocation, and to correct disk displacement. The suturing procedures employed by Israel, Tarro, and us differ in several ways. Israel's and Tarro's procedures both use a visible triangulation technique employing two cannulas for suturing. Israel's technique uses a 20-gauge injection needle, whereas Tarro's technique employs a semicircular suture needle. In both cases, manipulation is basically performed blindly. In our procedure, a suture needle is inserted directly into the joint and guided to the site of the suture while the needle tip is observed using an arthroscope. When suturing is complete, posterior disk shifting and anchoring are confirmed by arthroscopy.

Lasers were used in all patients reported in the present study. Although arthroscopic suturing was performed using a double-channel cannula, triangulation and a single-channel cannula could also have been used. As Israel describes, simple and accurate procedures are preferable to complex surgeries owing to the fact that the procedures are performed within the narrow confines of the TMJ cavity.[20]

SUMMARY

The application of the Nd:YAG laser in temporomandibular arthroscopic surgery proved to be useful in operations on the joint cavity. Treatment of hypermobility (subluxation), habitual dislocation, and anterior disk displacement of the TMJ had an overall success rate of over 92% after initial surgery. The arthroscopic suturing technique described herein features the insertion of a newly developed arthroscopic suture needle directly into the upper joint cavity. Using this needle in combination with a double-channel cannula makes this procedure relatively simple and much more accurate than single-channel cannula methods.

REFERENCES

1. Ohnishi, M. Arthroscopy of the temporomandibular joint [in Japanese]. Kokubyo Gakkai Zasshi (1975), 42:207–213.
2. Ohnishi, M. Arthroskopische Betrachtungen der Kiefergelenkshohle. In: Unfallverletzvagen des Kiefer-Gesichts-Bereichs: Acta Chirurgiae Maxillofacialis. Band 4. Leipzig: JA Barth (1979), 169–170.
3. Holmlund, A; Hellsing, G. Arthroscopy of the temporomandibular joint: An autopsy study. Int J Oral Surg (1985), 14:169–175.
4. Murakami, K; Ito, K. Arthroscopy of the temporomandibular joint. In: Watanabe, M, ed. Arthroscopy of Small Joints. Tokyo: Igaku-Shoin (1985), 128–139.
5. Goss, AN; Bosanquet, AG. Temporomandibular joint arthroscopy. J Oral Maxillofac Surg (1986), 4:614–617.

6. Sanders, B. Arthroscopic surgery of the temporomandibular joint: Treatment of internal derangement with persistent closed lock. Oral Surg Oral Med Oral Pathol (1986), 62:361–372.

7. Engelke, W. Feinnadel-Arthroskopiebefunde bei pathologischen Veränderungen des Kiefergelenks. *In:* Fortschritte der Kiefer- und Gesichtschirurgie. Band XXXII. Stuttgart: George Thieme Verlag (1987), 49–52.

8. McCain, JP. Arthroscopy of the human temporomandibular joint. J Oral Maxillofac Surg (1988), 46:648–655.

9. Ohnishi, M. Arthroscopic surgery for hypermobility and recurrent mandibular dislocation. Oral Maxillofac Surg Clin N Am (1989), 1:154–163.

10. Kino, K; Ohnishi, M; Shioda, S; Ichijo, T. Morphological observation on the inner surface of the temporomandibular joint: Histological investigation relating to the arthroscopic findings in the upper cavity [in Japanese]. Jpn J Oral Surg (1981), 27:1379–1389.

11. Ohnishi, M; Nakayama, E; Ohtsuki, K. Clinical evaluation of double-contrast computed tomography of the temporomandibular joint [in Japanese] (English abstract). Jpn J Oral Maxillofac Surg (1989), 35:155–167.

12. Ohnishi, M. Arthroscopy and arthroscopic surgery. *In:* Norman, J.E., Bramley, P, eds. Colour Atlas and Textbook of the Temporomandibular Joint Pathology and Surgery. London: Wolfe Publishing Co. (1990), 110–125.

13. Ohnishi, M. Newly designed needle scope system for the arthroscopic surgery by double-channel sheath method [in Japanese] (English abstract). J Jpn Soc TMJ (1989), 1:1–8.

14. Johnson, L. Diagnostic and Surgical Arthroscopy: The Knee and Other Joints. St. Louis: CV Mosby Co. (1981), 3–4.

15. Ozenis, P. Development of modern arthroscopic techniques, fundamentals of endoscopes, basic equipment for diagnosis and surgery. *In:* Parisien, JS, ed. Arthroscopic Surgery. New York: McGraw-Hill Book Co. (1988), 47–66.

16. Whipple, TI; Caspari, RB; Meyers, JF. Arthroscopic laser meniscectomy in a gas medium. Arthroscopy (1985), 1:1.

17. Smith, JB; Nance, TA. Laser energy in arthroscopic surgery. *In:* Parisien, JS, ed. Arthroscopic Surgery. New York: McGraw-Hill Book Co. (1988), 325–330.

18. Inoue, K. Arthroscopic laser surgery. *In:* Itami, Y, ed. Arthroscopic Diagnosis and Arthroscopic Surgery [in Japanese]. Tokyo: Kanehara Publishing Co. (1986), 187–197.

19. Ohnishi, M; Kanbayashi, H, Yaneyama, Y. Arthroscopic laser surgery of the temporomandibular joint [in Japanese] (English abstract). Arthroscopy (1986), 11:1–4.

20. Israel, HA. Technique for placement of a discal traction suture during temporomandibular joint arthroscopy. J Oral Maxillofac Surg (1989), 47:311–313.

21. Tarro, AW. Arthroscopic treatment of anterior disc displacement: A preliminary report. J Oral Maxillofac Surg (1989), 47:353–358.

Fourteen

Arthroscopic Traction Suturing
Treatment of Internal Derangement by Arthroscopic Repositioning and Suturing of the Disk

TOSHIROU KONDOH, D.M.D., Ph.D.

The temporomandibular joint (TMJ) is one of the smallest joints of the body. It has a disk that is similar to the meniscus of the knee joint. The disk of the TMJ is captured on the condyle and accompanies the condyle during jaw movement.[1,2]

Internal derangement of the TMJ is defined as *disk displacement*[3,4] that can be described as occurring either with reduction or without reduction. The selection of treatment differs according to the type of disk displacement presented. Patients with disk displacement with reduction have almost always been treated by conservative splint therapy.[5,6] However, treatment of long-standing cases of clicking, late-opening clicking, or clicking accompanied by hypermobility has not been successful. In such difficult cases of clicking, more active repositioning therapy is needed to treat the displaced disk. In the past, patients with these disorders were treated by open surgical techniques, such as disk repositioning surgery.[7]

Arthroscopic suturing operations were developed for knee joint surgery to suture the meniscus and fixate cartilage grafting.[8–10] The use of arthroscopic suture operations for the treatment of the TMJ was reported in 1989 by Israel,[11] Tarro,[12] Ohnishi,[13] and Kondoh.[14] The work of these surgeons addressed discal traction suturing of the TMJ for the treatment of anterior disk displacement. In this chapter, we present some new traction suturing procedures for the treatment of patients with difficult forms of clicking.

Our procedure is characterized by the penetration of the suture thread into the disk and its passage through the disk into the upper and lower joint compartments. This is followed by the tying and the securing of the thread to the cartilage of the external auditory canal. The posterolateral discal traction forces are effective in treating anteromedial disk displacement. The purpose of this procedure is to actively reposition a displaced disk and to stabilize a repositioned disk. This operation is performed arthroscopically, because invasive open surgical techniques upon the joint are considerably less successful.

CHARACTERIZATION OF PATIENTS

Disk displacement with reduction (clicking) is categorized as *progression displacement*.[3] Early-opening clicking indicates minimum anterior displacement, intermediate clicking is indicative of a relatively more advanced condition, and late clicking is present in patients with the most advanced anterior displacement. Both early clicking and intermediate clicking are conditions that have developed relatively recently in a patient, whereas late clicking is almost always a long-

117

standing condition.[3] In late clicking patients the disk is severely displaced and the retrodiscal tissue is elongated. Moreover, the displaced disk in such a configuration may be deformed.[15] The frequency of disk deformation in patients with clicking is not as great as that in patients with closed-lock.[16] In some patients with late clicking, the displaced disk is not totally recaptured and clicking continues.[17]

Hypermobility is characterized by an excessive range of opening motions,[18] but it is difficult to establish which of these motions is abnormal.[19,20] The late-opening click may be accompanied by hypermobility of the condyle. Clinically, patients with this type of clicking are strongly resistant to various therapies. We should set conservative limits as to which forms of clicking can be treated efficiently.

PLANNING A TREATMENT PROGRAM

All cases of disk displacement with reduction are initially treated with conservative splint therapy. Although anterior repositioning appliances are recommended for early- or intermediate-opening clicking, it is impossible to use these appliances for the treatment of late-opening clicking or hypermobility with clicking. In the presence of these disorders we have used flat stabilization splints or pivoting splints on the affected side. Some patients showed an improvement in disk position; such improvement was manifested in the form of a progression from late-opening clicking to intermediate or early clicking. If an anterior repositioning appliance is used instead of either a pivot splint or a stabilization splint, lower and upper joint compartment distention may be effective in treating more severe forms of clicking. This distention technique requires a saline solution injection into the joint compartment and the subsequent pumping of this solution.[21] The injection of a hyaluronic acid solution into the upper joint compartment may also be effective in decreasing articular surface friction.[22]

The distention or lubrication therapies described above aid in the conservative repositioning or the improvement of disk position. Unfortunately, these conservative therapies have not proved to be effective in treating most cases of long-standing clicking or advanced clicking. We reevaluated our patients 4–6 months after the start of conservative therapies. Patients who showed no change or insufficient improvement were recommended for an arthroscopic traction suturing operation.

PREOPERATIVE IMAGING ANALYSIS

The morphology of the articular eminence and the glenoid fossa of the temporal bone and the condyle

were examined using plain film or tomography in the sagittal and the coronal planes. In patients with clicking, bone morphologic changes (e.g., osteophyte or resorptive lesions of the condyle and bone irregularity of the posterior slope of the eminence) may be detectable on plain film. We were impressed by the presence of a deeper glenoid fossa and a higher eminence in patients with more serious cases of clicking.[23] These factors may result in severely loud clicking in the late stage of condylar motion.

With the teeth in the intercuspal position, the location of the condyle in the fossa should be recorded on film. The more severe the posterosuperior position of the condyles, the more difficult it will be to reposition the disk. The condyle position at the time of the clicking should be recorded on a plain film or a lateral tomograph of the sagittal plane.

The position and configuration of the disk are determined by magnetic resonance imaging (MRI) or double-contrast arthrotomography.[23–25] The disk position should be recorded at the time of the clicking. At this time, the disk may be incompletely reduced.[17] In patients presenting with severe bone changes of the joint compartments, a severe posterosuperior position of the condyle, serious disk deformation, or disk perforation, arthroscopic traction suturing is not recommended as a treatment option.

ARTHROSCOPIC INSTRUMENTATION

Arthroscopic traction suturing is accomplished by double-puncturing the upper joint compartment. Two or more irrigation cannulas, blunt obturators, or sharp-edged trocars are needed for each puncture. An 18-gauge injection needle is inserted into the lower joint compartment and is used to pass the suture thread through the punctures. A common wide-range (30 degree) arthroscope is used. A conventional light source and TV monitoring system are also employed. Bladed nylon (3–0 or 2–0) or Gore-Tex (3–0) is recommended as the suture thread for disk traction.

ARTHROSCOPIC PUNCTURE TECHNIQUES

To puncture the lower joint compartment the injection needle should be inserted into the posterior recess of the compartment. First, the lateral pole of the condyle is palpated. The needle is then advanced to the lateral pole as a mark. Next, the mouth is opened and the condyle is moved slightly forward. The tip of the needle touches the back end of the condyle, after which the needle is inserted further into the posterior recess of the lower joint compartment.

When the lateral approach for arthroscopic cannula insertion is used, the irrigation cannula is usually inserted by means of an inferolateral approach to the upper joint compartment.[27] However, in arthroscopic traction suturing, the irrigation cannula is inserted at the medial area of the posterior slope of the articular eminence. It is advantageous to inspect the central portion of the disk surface via this insertion approach.

When the endaural approach is used the arthroscopic cannula serves as a portal for the surgical instruments.[28] The cannula is guided by the illumination of the arthroscope that is passed through the lateral cannula. The endaural cannula should be positioned on the lateral side of the meatus.

ARTHROSCOPIC SUTURING

The operation begins with the insertion of an 18-gauge injection needle into the lower joint compartment of the TMJ (Fig. 14–1). The insertion is con-

firmed by injecting saline solution into the lower joint compartment and by pumping the lower joint space. A lateral puncture approach is used for the first irrigation cannula of the arthroscope; a water outflow needle is then inserted into the upper joint compartment (see Fig. 14–1).

A second cannula is then inserted via the endaural approach into the upper joint compartment (Fig. 14–2). Next, the 18-gauge needle in the lower joint compartment (see Fig. 14–2A) is moved upward to penetrate the posterior portion of the disk. The needle then passes through the disk into the upper joint compartment (Fig. 14–3A).

Next, the suture thread is guided into the upper joint compartment and is passed through the needle (see Fig. 14–3A). The tip of the thread is inserted into the upper joint compartment and is located arthroscopically (see Fig. 14–3B). While in the arthroscopic field of view the tip of the thread is clasped using alligator forceps that have been passed through the endaural cannula (Fig. 14–4A). The suture thread is

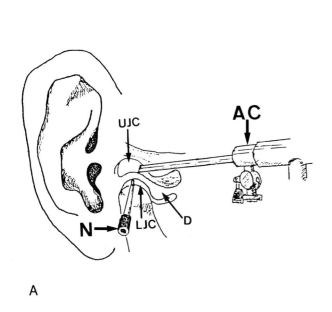
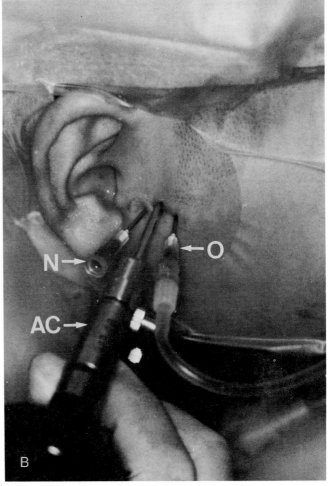

FIGURE 14–1. *A*—An 18-gauge injection needle is inserted into the lower joint space. An arthroscope is inserted into the upper joint space. *B*—The 18-gauge injection needle inserted into the lower joint space. (AC: arthroscope; N: 18-gauge injection needle; O: outflow needle; UJC: upper joint compartment; LJC: lower joint compartment; D: disk)

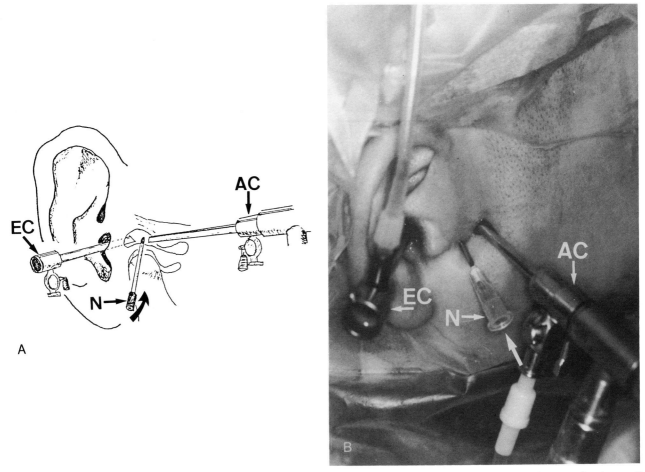

FIGURE 14–2. *A*—A second cannula (endaural cannula) is inserted into the upper joint space through an endaural approach. The needle penetrates the upper joint space. *B*—The needle penetrates the upper joint space. (AC: arthroscope; EC: endaural cannula; N: needle)

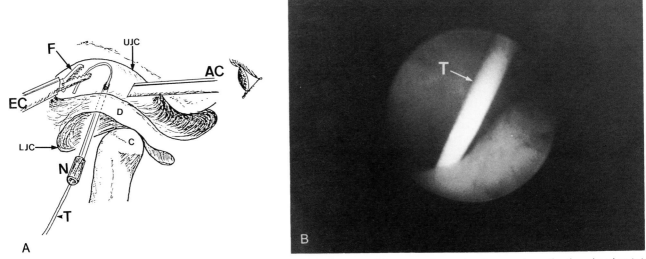

FIGURE 14–3. *A*—A suture thread passes through the needle and into the upper joint space. A grasping forceps clasps the thread end as it is viewed arthroscopically. *B*—Arthroscopic view of the penetrated suture thread in the upper joint space. (AC: arthroscope; EC: endaural cannula; N: needle; T: suture thread; F: grasping forceps; UJC: upper joint compartment; LJC: lower joint compartment; D: disk; C: condyle)

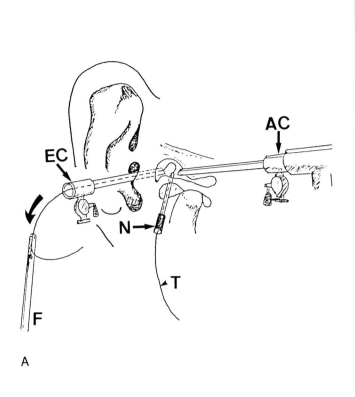

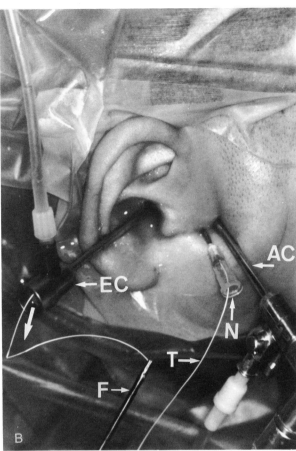

FIGURE 14–4. *A*—An end of thread is pulled out through the endaural cannula. *B*—An end of thread is pulled out through the endaural cannula. (F: grasping forceps; T: suture thread; EC: endaural cannula; N: needle; AC: endaural cannula)

then pulled out through the endaural cannula (see Fig. 14–4*B*), after which the endaural cannula is removed. At this point the suture thread has been passed through the lower joint compartment and has penetrated the disk (see Fig. 14–3*A*). The thread then travels through the upper joint compartment. Finally, the thread tip is pulled out through the cartilage wall of the extraauditory canal (Fig. 14–4*A*).

After this has been accomplished, the needle is pulled back into the lower joint compartment (Fig. 14–5*A*, 1). The needle tip is then rotated (Fig. 14–5*A*, 2) and pushed forward, penetrating the posterior wall of the lower joint compartment (Fig. 14–5*A*, 3) and passing through the endaural puncture area (see Fig. 14–5*B*). The thread is pulled out from the needle end (Fig. 14–6), and both thread ends are pulled out through the anterior wall of the extraauditory canal. The needle is then removed.

At this point the suture thread that has penetrated the disk has one of its ends passing through the lower joint compartment and the other passing through the upper joint compartment; both ends are exposed at the endaural wall (Fig. 14–7). Next, both thread ends are tugged back by the surgeon while an assistant

manipulates the mandible (see Fig. 14–7). The traction force is lateroposterior. The absence of clicking is confirmed by repeated manipulation. After manipulation is completed, the suture thread is tied to the cartilage of the extraauditory canal, and the disk is secured by the embedded suture. The operation is completed by suturing the skin surrounding the endaural wound and by embedding the suture thread.

POSTOPERATIVE PATIENT CARE

A stabilization splint should be worn by the patient when he or she awakes from anesthesia as the posterior intercuspal position may be raised slightly on the treated side of the jaw. This occlusal instability is a short-term phenomenon; however, it may cause a recurrence of disk displacement. Patients in our study were instructed to wear the splint all day for 3 weeks after the surgery. One month after surgery the patients were instructed to wear the splint while sleeping or as much as possible.

All patients displayed limited mouth opening for 3 weeks after surgery and were unable to eat solid food

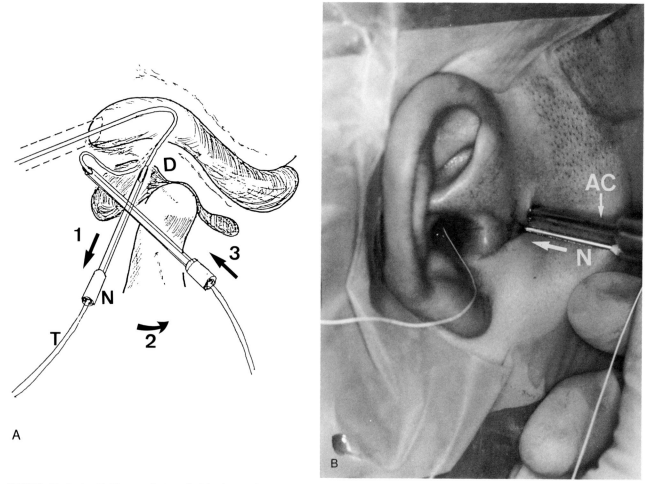

FIGURE 14–5. *A*—(1) The needle is pulled back into the lower joint space. (2) The needle is moved to the endaural puncture area. (3) The needle penetrates the endaural puncture area. *B*—The needle penetrates the endaural wall. (AC: arthroscope; N: needle; T: suture thread; D: disk)

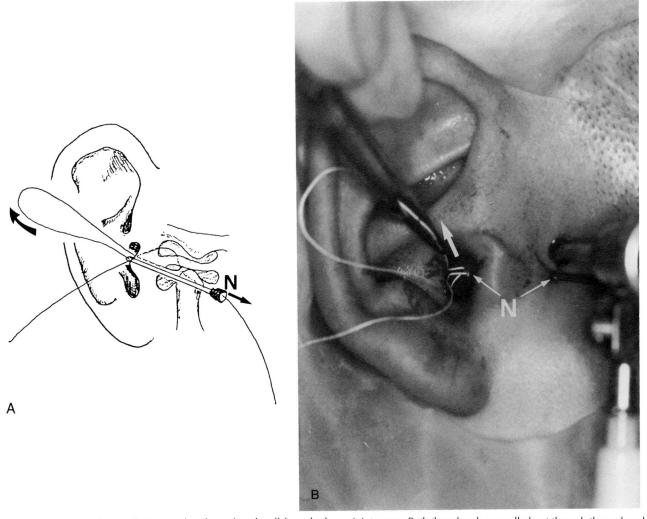

FIGURE 14–6. *A*—The needle is passed to the endaural wall from the lower joint space. Both thread ends are pulled out through the endaural wall. *B*—The other end of the thread is pulled out from the needle. (N: needle)

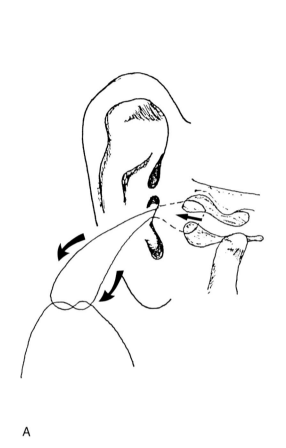

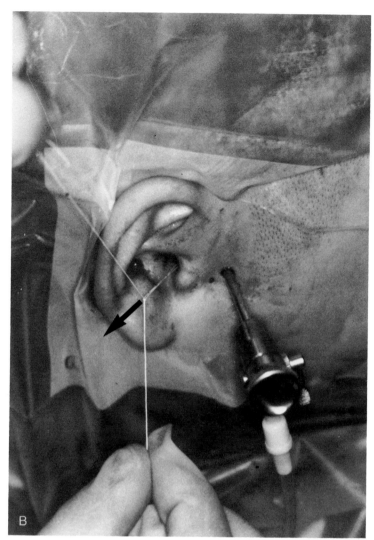

FIGURE 14–7. *A*—The suture threads are tied and pulled back for traction. *B*—The suture thread tugs back the disk.

for 1–2 weeks. The range of mouth opening motion increases after surgery such that one month postoperatively the mouth opening has increased to normal range in almost all patients. All patients were forbidden to passively open their mouths for 3 weeks after the procedure.

INITIAL CLINICAL EXPERIENCE WITH THE ARTHROSCOPIC SUTURING TECHNIQUE

We performed the described procedure on 10 patients with difficult clicking. The age of the patients ranged from 20 to 38 years, with a mean age of 26.4 years. The patient group comprised nine females and one male (Table 14–1). The preoperative diagnoses included three joints with late-opening clicking and seven hypermobile joints with clicking. Functional joint pain or clicking pain was observed preoperatively in three cases.

In the patients with hypermobility with clicking, the maximum opening (interincisal distance) had a range of 56–62 mm, with a mean of 58.9 mm. The interincisal opening in clicking-only patients had a range of 50–58 mm, with a mean of 53.7 mm. In the cases of late-opening clicking the mean interincisal opening was 46.3 mm. The duration of subjective patient symptoms ranged from 5 to 36 months, with a mean of 15.2 months.

Three of the ten patients had been treated for TMJ disorders at other clinics or hospitals. All of the patients had been treated with conservative therapies in our department for about 4–6 months prior to the surgery. The preoperative clicking of all patients was both severe and loud.

TABLE 14–1. DIAGNOSTIC PROFILE OF TEN PATIENTS (TEN JOINTS) PRIOR TO ARTHROSCOPIC SUTURING

Patient	Patient Age	Patient Sex	Affected TMJ* (Right or Left)	Diagnosis	Presence (+) or Absence (−) of Functional Joint Pain	Maximum Mouth Opening (Maximum Opening at Click)	Duration of Symptoms
1	23	Female	Right	Late clicking	−	45(43) mm	24 months
2	20	Male	Right	Hypermobility with clicking	−	56(50) mm	11 months
3	25	Female	Left	Hypermobility with clicking	−	60(56) mm	5 months
4	26	Female	Right	Hypermobility with clicking	+	60(50) mm	14 months
5	26	Female	Right	Hypermobility with clicking	−	62(58) mm	12 months
6	25	Female	Right	Hypermobility with clicking	−	58(54) mm	6 months
7	37	Female	Right	Late clicking	+	48(44) mm	36 months
8	38	Female	Right	Late clicking	+	46(44) mm	24 months
9	21	Female	Right	Hypermobility with clicking	−	58(52) mm	8 months
10	23	Female	Left	Hypermobility with clicking	−	58(56) mm	12 months

*Temporomandibular joint.

CLINICAL RESULTS

Clicking. In seven of ten joints, the clicking entirely disappeared after surgery. In two joints the clicking subsequently recurred 1–2 weeks after surgery. The two patients who experienced recurrence had preoperative diagnoses of hypermobility with clicking and late-opening clicking respectively (Table 14–2; see also Table 14–1).

Range of Opening Motion. In all patients diagnosed with hypermobility with clicking, the maximum opening decreased after surgery. The postoperative mean maximum opening was 48 mm, with a range of 44–54 mm. In the patients with late-opening clicking, maximum opening did not change significantly, with the mean maximum opening being 45 mm.

Functional Pain or Tenderness. Functional pain or tenderness of the affected joints was observed in three joints prior to surgery (see Table 14–1). This pain and tenderness disappeared in all joints postoperatively. However, postoperative pain or tenderness appeared in other patients (patients Nos. 3 and 9). These postoperative symptoms were very slight, and functional disturbance did not occur (see Table 14–2).

IMAGING FINDINGS AFTER ARTHROSCOPIC SUTURING

The disk position and disk configuration of all patients was analyzed by MRI prior to surgery. All joints were diagnosed to have anterior disk displacement with reduction. In patient No. 10 the disk was folded (Fig. 14–8). In patients Nos. 1 and 7 the disks were incompletely reduced after clicking. Postoperatively, six patients showed improved disk position and four patients failed to show any change in disk position (Fig. 14–9; see also Table 14–2).

SUMMARY

Arthroscopic surgery is a relatively new procedure for treating TMJ disorders. In the past, surgical repositioning for displaced disks was performed using open surgical techniques because it was not possible with arthroscopic surgery of the TMJ to actively reposition and stabilize the displaced disk. Arthroscopic surgery does have limitations associated with the instrumenta-

TABLE 14–2. POSTOPERATIVE RESULTS OF ARTHROSCOPIC SUTURING IN TEN PATIENTS (TEN JOINTS)

Patient	Status of Clicking	Maximum Mouth Opening (Maximum Opening at Click)	Presence (+) or Absence (−) of Functional Joint Pain	Status of Disk Position Based on MRI*
1	Recurred	45(40) mm	−	No change
2	Recurred	48(36) mm	−	No change
3	Disappeared	44(—) mm	+	No change
4	Disappeared	50(—) mm	−	Improved
5	Disappeared	54(—) mm	−	Improved
6	Disappeared	48(—) mm	−	Improved
7	Disappeared	46(—) mm	−	Improved
8	Disappeared	44(—) mm	−	Improved
9	Disappeared	46(—) mm	+	No change
10	Disappeared	46(—) mm	−	Improved

*Magnetic resonance imaging.

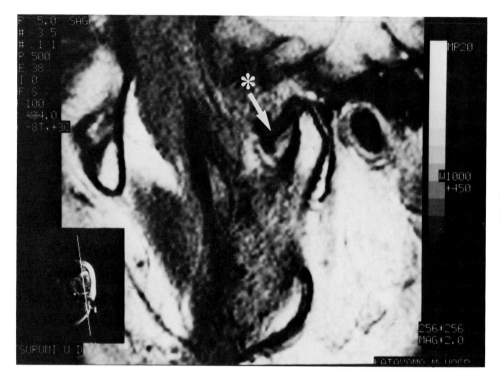

FIGURE 14–8. A preoperative magnetic resonance imaging (MRI). In the closed position, the disk was displaced anteriorly and folded. (*: disk folding)

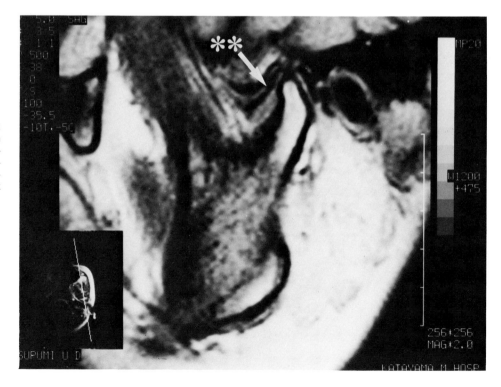

FIGURE 14–9. Postoperative MRI (the same case as in Fig. 14–8). In the closed position, the disk position was improved and the presence of disk folding had disappeared. (**: absence of disk folding)

tion and surgical technology it requires. However, arthroscopic surgery is much less invasive than open surgical techniques and is therefore much less traumatic.

Our discussion of the arthroscopic traction suturing technique is still incomplete. As postoperative care and occlusal stabilization improve, the number of good postoperative outcomes is expected to increase. However, surgical disk repositioning should be performed only in those patients for whom the surgical procedure promises the greatest benefit.

REFERENCES

1. Bell, WE. Temporomandibular Disorders. Chicago: Year Book Medical Publishers, Inc. (1990), 71–81.
2. Howerton, DW; Zysset, M. Anatomy of the temporomandibular joint and related structures with surgical anatomic considerations. Oral Maxillofac Surg Clin N Am (1989), 1:229–247.
3. Farrar, WB; McCarty, Jr., W. A Clinical Outline of Temporomandibular Joint Diagnosis and Treatment. Montgomery, Alabama: Walker Printing Co. (1983), 53–56.
4. Ad Hoc Study Group on TMJ Meniscus Surgery. 1984 Criteria for TMJ Meniscus Surgery. American Association of Oral and Maxillofacial Surgery, Chicago, 1984.
5. Clark, GT. Treatment of jaw clicking with temporomandibular repositioning: Analysis of 25 cases. J Craniomandib Pract (1984), 2:264–270.
6. Anderson, CG; Schulte, JK. Comparative study of two treatment methods for internal derangement of the temporomandibular joint. J Prosthet Dent (1985), 53:392–397.
7. Dolwick, MF; Sanders, B. TMJ Internal Derangement and Arthrosis. Surgical Atlas. St. Louis: CV Mosby Co. (1985), 142–180.
8. Stone, RG. Peripheral Detachment of the menisci of the knee: A preliminary report. Orthop Clin North Am (1979), 10:643–657.
9. DeHaven, KE. Peripheral meniscal repair: An alternative to meniscectomy. Orthop Transact (1981), 5:399–400.
10. Hendler, RC. Arthroscopic meniscal repair surgical techniques. Clin Orthop (1984), 190:163–169.
11. Israel, HA. Technique for placement of a discal traction suture during temporomandibular joint arthroscopy. J Oral Maxillofac Surg (1989), 47:311–313.
12. Tarro, AW. Arthroscopic treatment of anterior disk displacement: A preliminary report. J Oral Maxillofac Surg (1989), 47:353–358.
13. Ohnishi, M. Arthroscopic surgery for hypermobility and recurrent mandibular dislocation. Oral Maxillofac Surg Clin N Am (1989), 1:153–164.
14. Kondoh, T. Arthroscopic traction suture for clicking and hypermobility of the temporomandibular joint. Abstract presented at the Seventy-second Annual Meeting and Scientific Sessions of the American Association of Oral and Maxillofacial Surgery. September 1990.
15. Westesson, PL; Bronstein, SL. Internal derangement of the temporomandibular Joint: Morphologic description with correlation to joint function. Oral Surg (1985), 59:323–331.
16. Westesson, PL. Double-contrast arthrotomography of the temporomandibular joint: Introduction of an arthrographic technique for visualization of the disc and articular surfaces. J Oral Maxillofac Surg (1983), 41:163–172.
17. Eriksson, L; Westesson, PL. Temporomandibular joint sounds in patients with disc displacement. Int J Oral Surg (1985), 14:428–436.
18. Merrill, RG. Mandibular dislocation and hypermobility. Oral Maxillofac Surg Clin N Am (1989), 1:399–413.
19. Mezitis, M; Rallis, G. The normal range of mouth opening. J Oral Maxillofac Surg (1989), 47:1028–1029.
20. Bates, RE; Stewart, CM. The relationship between internal derangements of the TMJ and systemic joint laxity. J Am Dent Assoc (1984), 109:446–447.
21. Murakami, K; Matsuki, M. Recapturing the persistent anteriorly displaced disc by mandibular manipulation after pumping and hydraulic pressure to the upper joint cavity of the temporomandibular joint. J Craniomandib Pract (1987), 5:17–24.
22. Kopp, S; Wenneberg, B; Haraldson, T; Carlsson, GE. The short-term effect of intra-articular injections of sodium hyaluronate and corticosteroid on temporomandibular joint pain and dysfunction. J Oral Maxillofac Surg (1985), 43:429–435.
23. Hall, MB; Gipps, CC. Association between the prominence of the articular eminence and displaced TMJ disks. J Craniomandib Pract (1985), 3:238–239.
24. Westesson, PL; Rolin, M. Diagnostic accuracy of double-contrast arthrotomography of the temporomandibular joint: Correlation with postmortem morphology. AJNR (1984), 5:463–468.
25. Hansson, LG; Westesson, PL. MR Imaging of the temporomandibular joint: Comparison of images of autopsy specimens made at 0.3T and 1.5T with anatomic cryosections. AJR (1989), 152:1241–1244.
26. Katzberg, RW. Temporomandibular joint imaging. Radiology (1989), 170:297–307.
27. Murakami, K; Ono, T. Temporomandibular joint arthroscopy by inferolateral approach. Int J Oral Maxillofac Surg (1986), 15:410–417.
28. Moses, JJ; Poker, ID. Temporomandibular joint arthroscopy: The endaural approach. Int J Oral Maxillofac Surg (1989), 18:347–351.

Fifteen

Arthroscopic Laser Procedures

A. THOMAS INDRESANO, D.M.D.
JON BRADRICK, D.D.S.

It has been our opinion that the delivery of laser energy through the arthroscope would be extremely beneficial for temporomandibular joint (TMJ) surgery. We have therefore undertaken a long-term research project to investigate this belief. Our project can be broken down into three phases. First, *in vitro* and acute studies were performed in order to assess the suitability of using a laser on the tissues in the joint and to assess the potential delivery systems (Fig. 15–1). Next, chronic studies were performed in order to assess laser wounds in the joint tissues and to study the ability of these tissues to heal (Fig. 15–2). Finally, a clinical model of adhesive capsulitis was developed and treated using a laser (Fig. 15–3).

Can laser energy be effectively utilized to treat TMJ disorders? A classification of available lasers and their properties was made with the goal of identifying the ideal laser for this use (Fig. 15–4 and Table 15–1). The beam of the ideal laser for the arthroscopic treatment of the TMJ must be transmissible via a fiberoptic light cable (Fig. 15–5). It must be able to cut and coagulate, and its beam should be visible to the eye so that it may be easily and safely aimed. Finally, it should not damage distant structures or areas outside the field of surgery. Although no laser in our study met all of these criteria, those that fulfilled the most were the neodymium-yttrium-aluminum-garnet (Nd:YAG) laser and the KTP-532. The availability of an Nd:YAG laser at our institution simplified our choice.

Difficulty in aiming and the possibility of local injury outside of the target field were two areas of concern presented by the Nd:YAG laser. The Nd:YAG laser must be focused using an aiming light because the beam it produces is invisible to the human eye. This shortcoming might lead to questions as to whether the laser is active and as a result might require some compromise in technique to ensure that the beam of the active laser can be distinguished from that of the inactive. As the use of the Nd:YAG laser in the bowel has been shown to cause distant injury, we remained alert to the possibility of damage to areas outside the surgical field.[1] The second phase of the study was designed specifically to stress the limits of safety when

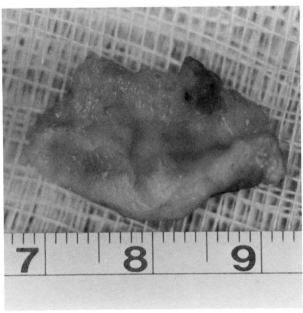

FIGURE 15–1. Laser energy imparted to canine disk *in vitro*.

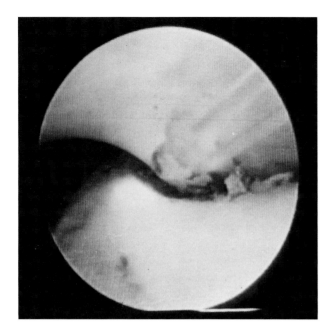

FIGURE 15–2. Arthroscopic view of a laser wound as it is formed.

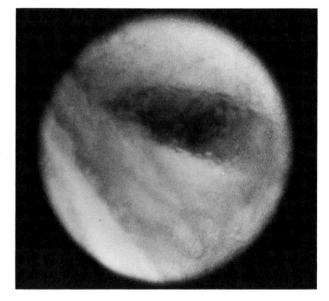

FIGURE 15–3. Arthroscopic view of a model of adhesive capsulitis.

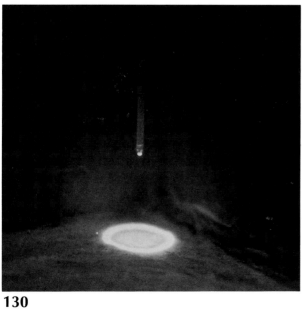

FIGURE 15–4. Aiming light.

TABLE 15–1. SPECIFICATIONS AND APPLICATIONS OF VARIOUS LASERS

Type	Wavelength	Power Requirement (in Watts)	Adaptability to Fiberoptic Use	Compatible with a Water Medium	Range of Use
CO_2	10,600 nm	100 W	Difficult	No	Cutting
Erbium-YAG	2940 nm	50 W	Difficult	No	Cutting
Holmium:YAG	2150 nm	50 W	Difficult	No	Cutting
Multi.YAG	1440 nm	50 W	Yes	No	Cutting
	1320 nm	50 W	Yes	Yes	Coagulation
	1060 nm	100 W	Yes	Yes	Coagulation
Nd:YAG	1060 nm	100 W	Yes	Yes	Coagulation and Cutting
KTP-532	532 nm	20 W	Yes	Yes	Coagulation and Cutting
Argon	488 nm	15 W	Yes	Yes	Limited

using high energy levels to identify ways to prevent injury of distant tissues. Finally, the procedures in the first phase of the study were repeated using the KTP-532 laser. This was done so that the outcome of treatment using the KTP-532 laser could be compared with that of the Nd:YAG laser.

PHASE 1

In vitro studies were performed on canine TMJ tissues that were collected from animals being used for other purposes (Fig. 15–6). Various wound patterns, laser energy settings, and exposure times were used. The laser could be used in a contact or a noncontact mode. The cutting of tissues, including disk tissue, was performed. Shrinkage in overall tissue size was observed and could be correlated with changes in the intensity of laser energy applied (Fig. 15–7).

Acute animal studies focused on techniques of using the laser in combination with the arthroscope. The fiberoptic bundle was inserted into the canine TMJ cavity via an outflow cannula, making possible the application of laser energy to any portion of the joint. Arthroscopic laser surgery was then begun. Cutting, coagulating, débridement, and contact cutting were performed. Safety studies were conducted to determine the effect of passing the maximum available energy into the TMJ. It was evident at the outset that temperature was a very important factor, so a temperature study was also performed. The study showed the temperature at the laser target area to be very high for extremely short periods; however, the circulating fluid maintained the temperature well within the range of acceptability, even a few millimeters away from the target. Decreasing the fluid temperature did not result in any change, since circulation of the fluid was the main factor. This finding correlated well with the

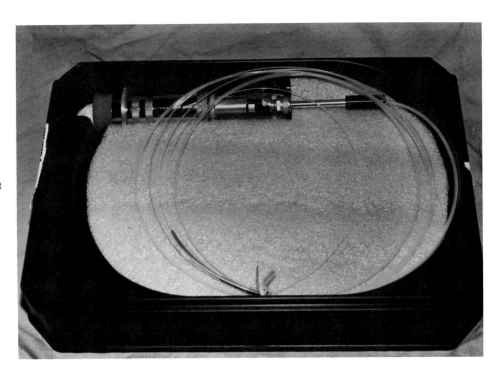

FIGURE 15–5. Fiberoptic light bundle.

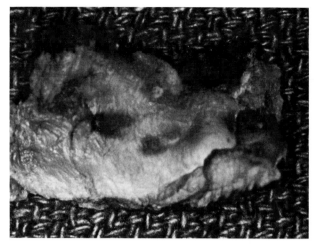

FIGURE 15–6. Excised canine disk.

findings of thermal studies of electrocautery in the TMJ. However, it was evident that long periods of laser exposure without adequate pauses during which fluid circulation could equalize temperatures were to be avoided.

The immediate effects in the fibrocartilaginous disk were similar to those reported following laser wounds to connective tissue in other parts of the body. On hematoxylin-and-eosin (H & E)–stained sections examined under low power, the noncontact wounds appeared as intense eosinophilic areas. The superior and the inferior surfaces of the disk were intact, with the deeper tissues being most affected. This indicates the Nd:YAG laser's ability to penetrate tissues and to produce a deep effect without surface vaporization. On higher magnification, the burned area showed a loss of the normal linear, layered fibrocartilage architecture and displayed disorganization of fiber patterns. The background was globular and homogeneous. Nuclei were small and pyknotic, with the nucleic lacunae

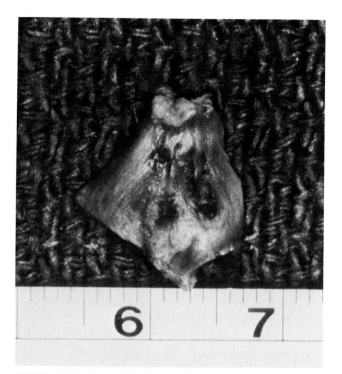

FIGURE 15–7. Canine disk showing shrinkage after laser wounds.

nearly empty (Fig. 15–8). The contact burns appeared as circular or elliptic punched-out tissue defects. Three distinct zones were seen around the cleft: (1) a thin and densely eosinophilic coagulum zone; (2) an irregular and hypodense zone of cavitation with globular areas of vacuolization; and (3) an eosinophilic and homogeneous acidophilic zone containing scattered pyknotic nuclei. Masson's trichrome stained the non-contact laser burn intensely red, but the surrounding area failed to take up the stain and remained clear. The same change in fibrocartilage architecture as found in the H & E–stained sections was observed, but the

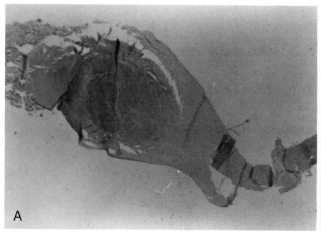
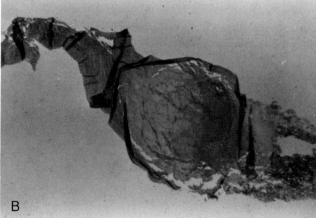

FIGURE 15–8. Histologic changes after noncontact laser wounds. A—Hematoxylin and eosin (H & E)–stained section. B—Masson's trichrome–stained section.

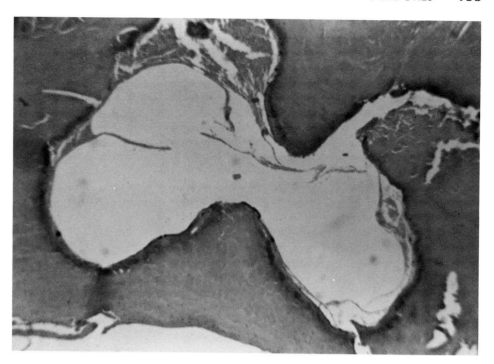

FIGURE 15–9. Histologic changes after contact laser burn. H & E–stained section.

globular disorganization was replaced by disorganized strands separating the globular background material (Fig. 15–9). Contact burns were able to ablate the disk or to cut through it, whereas noncontact energy could be used to coagulate fibrillation or finer adhesions.

PHASE 2

The second part of the project addressed the healing of laser wounds in the TMJ. Animals underwent surgery involving the use of a laser arthroscope prototype that had a coaxial port, which allowed the passage of a 400-μm fiber (Fig. 15–10). Arthroscopy was repeated at 1- and 2-week intervals. At rearthroscopy sections were collected for histologic examination.

Laser wounds of the synovial structures healed within 1 week, but disk wounds made by contact were not healed at 2 weeks (Fig. 15–11). Damage found in the condylar cartilage cap in one dog that underwent disk cuts stressed the potential for distant damage within the joint (Fig. 15–12). As a part of this study, the peak energy levels of the laser were used to create both contact and noncontact wounds in all parts of the joint. This was done in order to determine the safety parameters of the system. It was shown that the bony walls of the TMJ confine and obtund the energy beam. The dense connective tissues of the capsule perform the same function. The laser energy that can be applied through a 400–600-μm fiber cannot cause distant destruction. Local destruction within the joint is certainly possible, and efforts should be made to avoid it. It must be noted that the potential for distant injury exists, especially when the laser is in the noncontact mode. This potential must be assessed with every increase in fiber size to allow for possible increases in laser energy application.

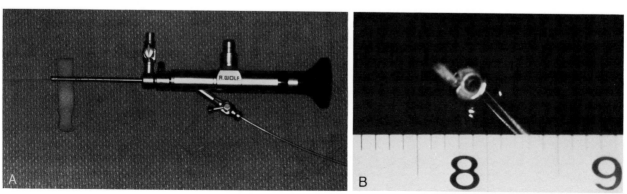

FIGURE 15–10. Laser arthroscope. (Wolfe Inc., Chicago, Ill)

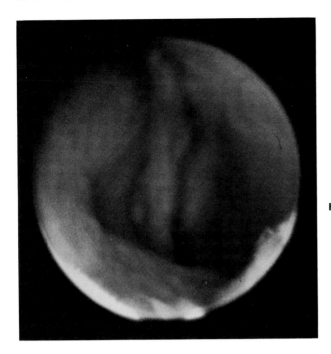

FIGURE 15–11. Laser wound showing healing.

FIGURE 15–12. Laser wound autopsy specimen showing local damage to adjacent tissues.

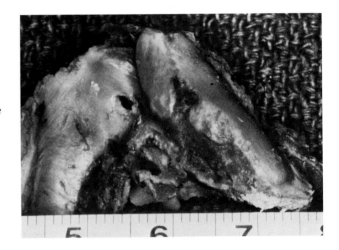

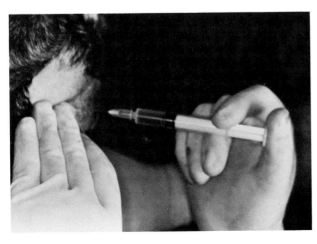

FIGURE 15–13. Injection of a canine temporomandibular joint with a 5% morrhuate sodium solution.

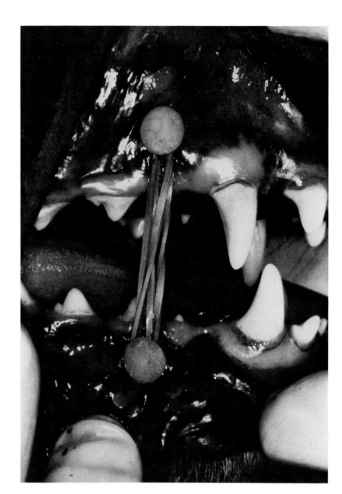

FIGURE 15–14. Canine intermaxillary fixation.

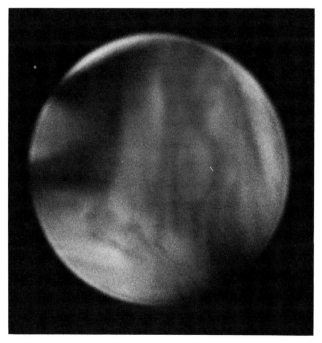

FIGURE 15–15. Joint adhesions.

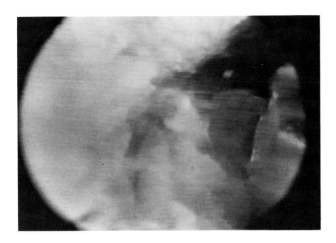

FIGURE 15–16. Débridement of adhesions using a neodymium-yttrium-aluminum-garnet laser.

PHASE 3

How can the laser be best used in the TMJ? The third part of the project addressed this question by studying a clinical situation. Adhesive capsulitis, a commonly encountered condition, was chosen for simulation. Canine TMJs were injected with a 5% morrhuate sodium solution (Fig. 15–13). The dogs were held in intermaxillary fixation (elastic traction between direct bone screws) for 2 weeks (Fig. 15–14). The animals were to be inspected arthroscopically at weekly intervals, but it was soon evident that 1 week proved to be sufficient to achieve mild to moderate adhesive capsulitis (Fig. 15–15).

The canine TMJs were débrided using the laser arthroscope. Follow-up continued for 2–4 weeks. Arthroscopy was repeated at weekly intervals. Débride-

ment of the joints was easy to perform using the Nd:YAG laser (Fig. 15–16). Healing progressed normally after an initial inflammatory response, with full healing found at 4 weeks (Fig. 15–17). The joints healed well and showed no signs of the return of adhesions (Fig. 15–18). The degree of healing without fibrosis was impressive when compared with that occurring after the use of mechanical débridement in other situations. We propose that a direct comparison of the two modalities should be performed in the future.

It is our belief that sufficient evidence now exists to incorporate the Nd:YAG laser into the TMJ arthroscopic armamentarium. Although we did not replicate each step using the KTP-532 laser, it is believed that this laser should perform similarly to the Nd:YAG laser, and therefore can serve as an alternative.

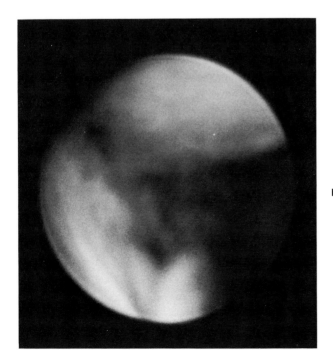

FIGURE 15–17. Healing after laser débridement.

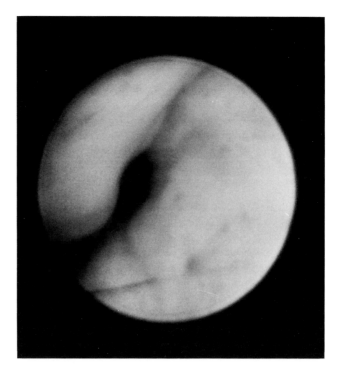

FIGURE 15–18. Completed healing after laser débridement.

REFERENCES

1. Schroder, T; Brackett, K; Joffe, SN. An experimental study of the effects of electrocautery and various lasers on gastrointestinal tissue. Surgery (1987), 101:691–697.
2. Bradrick, JP; Eckhauser, ML; Indresano, AT. Morphologic and histologic changes in canine temporomandibular joint tissues following arthroscopic guided neodymium:YAG laser exposure. J Oral Maxillofac Surg (1989), 47:1177–1181.
3. Indresano, AT; Bradrick, JP; Eckhauser, ML. Nd:YAG laser arthroscopy of the temporomandibular joint. Lecture presented at the Eighth Congress of the International Society for Laser Surgery and Medicine, Taipei, Taiwan, November 1989.
4. Ohnishi, M. Arthroscopic surgery for hypermobility and recurrent mandibular dislocation. Oral Maxillofac Surg Clin N Am (1989), 1:153–164.

PART 4

Research

Sixteen

Development of the Canine Model for Investigative Temporomandibular Joint Arthroscopy

A. THOMAS INDRESANO, D.M.D.
JON BRADRICK, D.D.S.

The development and the acceptance of techniques of temporomandibular joint (TMJ) arthroscopy have progressed at a rapid pace, yet many of the techniques have failed to evolve from sound animal research models prior to their implementation in human patients. Contributing to this lack of investigation may be the absence of a suitable animal model.

REQUIREMENTS OF ANIMAL MODELS

Previous TMJ arthroscopy research models were limited to rabbits,[1-3] sheep,[4,5] and human cadavers.[6] The ideal animal model for investigative TMJ arthroscopy must possess several essential qualities. The animal should be inexpensive to acquire and maintain. The animal's TMJs should correlate with human TMJs with respect to their anatomy, volume, histology, and function. The induction and the maintenance of anesthesia for the animal should be simple and require a minimum of agents and equipment. Animal husbandry should be simple, not require accessory equipment, and involve procedures that enable the majority of research facilities to house the particular animal. The animal should be readily available and simple to obtain.

Last, the animal should be considered ethically acceptable for research purposes to the local contingent of animal welfare groups (Table 16–1).

The initial investigations involving human TMJ arthroscopy were performed on cadavers.[6] These studies were invaluable for defining anatomic landmarks and evaluating instrumentation; however, dynamic studies of the responses of living tissue require an animal model.

TABLE 16–1. PREVIOUS TMJ* ANIMAL MODELS

Suitability Factors	Animal	
	Rabbit	*Sheep*
Cost	Inexpensive	Expensive†
Human correlation	TMJ smaller than the human TMJ	TMJ similar to the human TMJ
Ease of anesthetization	Difficult; similar to a pediatric case	Routine
Husbandry	Simple	Special facilities required†
Availability	Readily available‡	Not readily available†
Ethical acceptability	No problems	No problems

*Temporomandibular joint.
†Depending on the location (e.g., does not apply in Australia).
‡Depending on the strain.

California albino rabbits weighing approximately 8–10 lbs were utilized in the late 1970s by Hilsabeck and Laskin.[1] However, in a later study, Williams and Laskin chose instead to use giant Flemish rabbits weighing 16–20 lbs because the smaller rabbits were inadequate as TMJ arthroscopic models.[2] The New Zealand white rabbit strain, popular for open TMJ surgical models, weighs 6–11 lbs and would therefore be as unsuitable as the California albino species as an arthroscopic model. The lack of additional literature reporting the use of the rabbit as a TMJ arthroscopic model reflects the technical limitation of this animal's small joint space or is evidence of the difficulties encountered in obtaining the larger strains.

Bosanquet and Goss first described use of the Australian Merino sheep as a model for investigative TMJ surgery in 1987, and they discussed its use as an arthroscopic model in 1989.[4,5] The larger joint space and extensive range of motion of the ruminant sheep TMJ provided an excellent research model similar in size and anatomy to the human TMJ. Merino sheep are extremely plentiful and easily obtained in Australia; however, the utilization of sheep as TMJ research models has not been popular in the United States because of the unfeasibility of accommodating animals of their size at many hospital-based research facilities. Sheep have been utilized as acute teaching models at several continuing-education courses in TMJ arthroscopy in the United States. Nonhuman primates, although seemingly suitable anatomically, are prohibitively expensive.

Finally, it should be noted that mice and rats are too small to deserve consideration as TMJ arthroscopic models.

THE CANINE TMJ

Like the human TMJ, the canine temporomandibular articulation is divided into two spaces: the superior and the inferior. A thin, biconcave fibrocartilaginous disk divides the two spaces. The superior space is larger than the inferior, and the volume of the canine joint is similar to that of the human. The canine joint bony surfaces are lined with articulating cartilage, and a lateral capsular ligament attaches these surfaces to the condyle, the disk, and the temporal bone. Synovial tissue lines the peripheral aspects of each joint space and is concentrated in the extreme anterior and posterior aspects of the joint. The canine joint does not have a posterior attachment as does its human counterpart. The canine disk is attached at its medial aspect to the base of the temporal bone by a very strong tendon. This is an exceptionally prominent feature, and represents a landmark in the arthroscopy of the canine superior joint space.

The canine TMJ has a very large retroarticular process that forms the posterior border of the joint. This process is easily palpable and serves as a critical landmark for arthroscopic puncture. The mandibular condyle is greatly elongated mediolaterally and does not present with intercondylar angulation as it does in humans. This reflects the uniaxial rotational function of the carnivore temporomandibular articulation. Very few translational, protrusive, or lateral excursions are possible in this type of joint architecture.[7]

It has been our experience that canine anesthesia is the easiest form of animal anesthesia; however, it is best accomplished with an assistant. The morning feeding is withheld from the animals, but water is always available for them preoperatively. Twenty-five mg/kg of intravenous sodium pentobarbital (Nembutal, Abbott Laboratories, Chicago) is injected into the cephalic vein, found on the anterior and medial surface of the foreleg distal to the elbow. Shaving and antiseptic preparation should precede the venipuncture. The anesthetic provides about 2 hours of surgical anesthesia. Local anesthesia with epinephrine is infiltrated over the TMJ and into the superior joint space for analgesia and hemostasis. The use of neuromuscular blocking agents and mechanical ventilation has not been found to be necessary for this procedure; however, intubation with a large oral endotracheal tube is necessary for airway protection. The emergence from sodium pentobarbital anesthesia is slow; when the dog in a chronic study is returned to its cage a recovery time of 3–4 hours should be expected.

THE CROSSBITE DISTRACTION TECHNIQUE

The canine TMJ, like the human TMJ, has limited space in which to insert an arthroscope. To facilitate human arthroscopy, a protrusive maneuver is employed to access the superior joint space from the posterior approach. This maneuver is not effective in the canine TMJ owing to its limited range of motion. We have developed a technique of sustained, extreme lateral excursion that permits superior joint space arthroscopy in the canine TMJ. We term this maneuver the *crossbite distraction technique*. The materials required for the technique include a local anesthetic containing vasoconstrictors, wire cutters, a wire twister, a small mandibular awl, and heavy-gauge stainless steel wire (0.022–0.024 inch in diameter). Following the induction of general anesthesia, the local anesthetic is infiltrated into the maxillary and the mandibular buccal vestibules located opposite the canine teeth. Additional anesthetic is injected into the midline of the palate located between the canines, through both nares into the nasal septum, and into the anterior midline of the floor of the mouth.

If arthroscopy is to be performed on the *right* canine TMJ, a small mandibular awl is passed through the *left* external nares along the nasal floor to a point between the canines in the midline and next to the nasal septum. The awl is then directed into the oral cavity through the large left canine incisive foramen (Fig. 16–1). A heavy stainless steel wire is then secured to the awl in the oral cavity. The wire and awl are then retracted back into the nasal cavity. Next, the tip of the awl is directed over the piriform aperture until it emerges into the maxillary left buccal vestibule anterior to the left canine (Fig. 16–2). The wire is then released from the awl, and the awl is removed from the nasal cavity. The awl is then directed from an external submental approach into the right mandibular buccal vestibule, emerging distal to the mandibular right canine. The wire that emerges from the palatal aspect of the incisive foramen is then secured to the awl in the mandibular right buccal vestibule. The awl and the wire are then directed under the mandible to emerge in the midline of the floor of the mouth. The location of the wire at the floor of the mouth is determined by the mandibular symphysis, which projects posteriorly a considerable distance. The circumbimaxillary wire is now in place.

Next, the mandible is forcefully distracted laterally to the left, and the maxillary left buccal vestibule wire is secured to the mandibular wire exiting from the floor of the mouth using a wire twister. Normally, the maxillary palatal surfaces of the canine first molar

articulate with the buccal surfaces of the mandibular first molar. The length, the large surface area, and the angulation of these surfaces are used as an inclined plane to guide the mandible into a left crossbite. The lingual surface of the mandibular first molar should now oppose the buccal surface of the maxillary first molar. The jaws are then forcibly closed together. The buccal crossbite relationship of the left first molars will cause extreme left deviation of the mandible as it is closed. The circumbimaxillary wire is then twisted to secure the left anterior maxilla to the right mandibular body. When the procedure is done correctly, the right mandibular canine should appear aligned with the maxillary midline (Fig. 16–3). The extreme left deviation of the mandible serves to displace the right mandibular condyle anteriorly, thereby enlarging the right posterior aspect of the superior joint space. This technique seems to work better on dogs that are dolichocephalic (having a long, anteroposterior facial projection).

ARTHROSCOPY TECHNIQUE

Following distraction of the canine TMJ undergoing arthroscopy, the area over the joint is shaved and prepared. Palpation of the zygomatic arch posteriorly reveals a prominent preauricular cleft where the posterior aspect of the zygomatic arch takes an abrupt medial turn. This represents the posterolateral aspect of the TMJ. Further palpation of this area reveals the

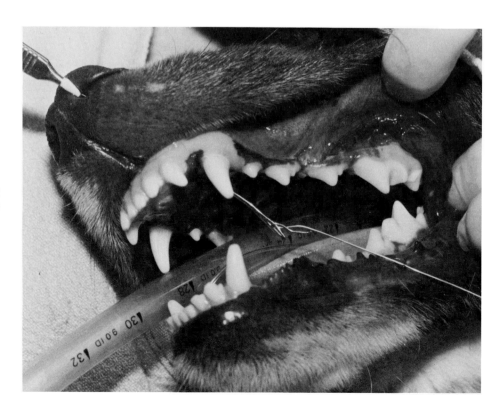

FIGURE 16–1. Initial passage of the awl through the canine incisive foramen.

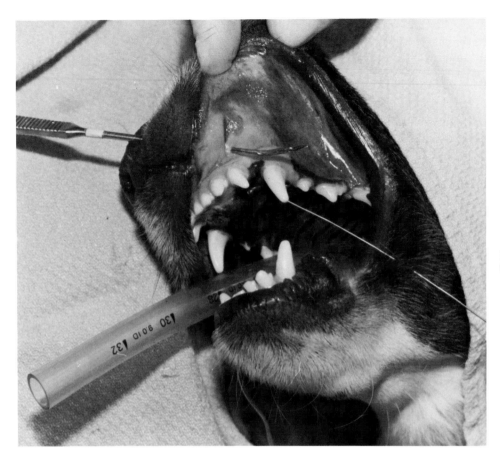

FIGURE 16–2. Wire passage from the nasal cavity into the oral cavity.

FIGURE 16–3. Completed cross-bite distraction with the mandibular right alveolus wired to the maxillary left alveolus. Note the induced crossbite of the left molars (*arrow*) with their inclined planes guiding the distraction of the *right* temporomandibular joint (TMJ).

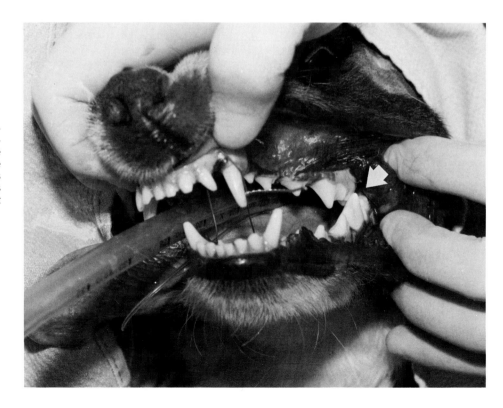

curved retroarticular process and the lateral pole of the mandibular condyle. Movement of the condyle is not detected when the teeth are wired for distraction. A semilunar depression, which represents the superior joint space, can be felt inferiorly between the posterior aspect of the zygomatic arch and the retroarticular process. After a 2–3-mm incision is made *through the skin only*, the arthroscopic sheath with the sharp trocar is advanced through the lateral joint capsule. A distinctive "pop" similar to that occurring in human TMJ arthroscopy can be felt. After the bone is encountered in the glenoid fossa, the arthroscopic sheath and trocar must be redirected parallel to the coronal plane and perpendicular to the sagittal plane of the dog's head in order to achieve proper angular penetration into the superior joint space. Following placement of an irrigation outflow needle into either the anterior or the posterior aspect of the superior joint space and replacement of the trocar with an arthroscopic telescope and camera, TMJ arthroscopy may proceed as in a human patient.

The most important landmark to be identified in the superior joint space is the medial attachment of the disk. It is visible as a funnel-shaped tendon that disappears deep toward the posteromedial aspects of the compartment. The medial attachment of the disk divides the superior joint space into its anterior and posterior recesses, which are orientated at 90 degrees to each other. Caution should be exercised because the maxillary artery lies immediately medial to this

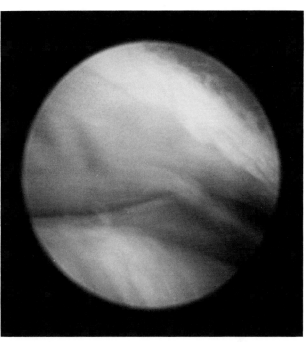

FIGURE 16–5. Arthroscopy of the canine left TMJ superior compartment. The view is more posterior than that shown in Figure 16–4.

attachment. We have encountered some spectacular hemorrhaging when using a fiber-guided laser in the area of the canine medial attachment.

Inspection of the posterior recess, proceeding in an inferior direction, reveals a thin, vascular synovial lining at the tip of the retroarticular process. Access to the anterior recess is not always possible as the

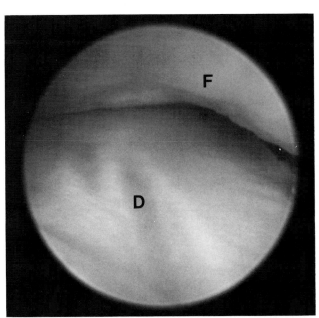

FIGURE 16–4. Arthroscopy of the canine left TMJ superior compartment. Here and in Figures 16–5 to 16–9 the orientation is as follows: anterior is to the left, posterior is to the right, superior is at the top of the picture, and inferior is at the bottom of the picture. (D: articulating disk; F: glenoid fossa)

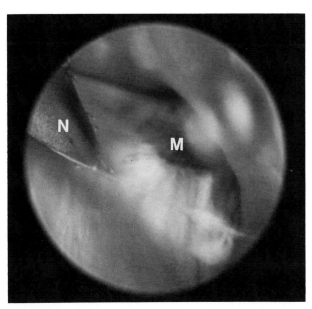

FIGURE 16–6. Arthroscopy of the canine left TMJ superior compartment. The view is more posterior than that shown in Figure 16–5. Note the medial attachment tapering toward the posteromedial aspects of the superior compartment. An 18-gauge outflow needle is visible in the field at the 10 o'clock position. (M: medial attachment; N: outflow needle)

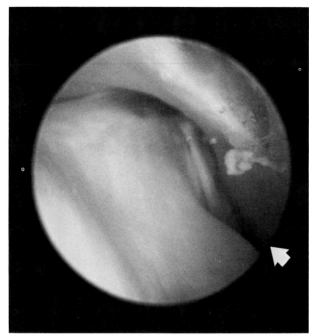

FIGURE 16–7. Arthroscopy of the canine left TMJ superior compartment. The view is more inferior than that shown in Figure 16–6. Note the medial disk attachment. The irregular area on the glenoid fossa from the 12 o'clock to 3 o'clock position is the iatrogenic trauma from the initial joint entry. Note the start of posterior recess (arrow). (M: medial disk attachment)

crossbite distraction technique may force the condyle against the anterior part of the glenoid fossa. In many cases, however, it is possible to position the arthroscope in the anterior recess or to direct its angle of

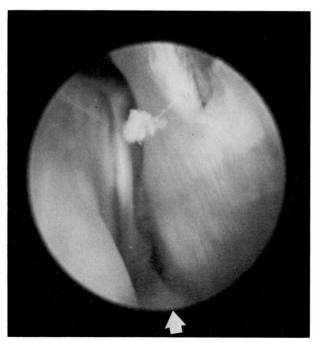

FIGURE 16–8. Arthroscopy of the canine left TMJ superior compartment. The view is more inferior than that shown in Figure 16–7. (M: medial attachment; *arrow:* posterior recess)

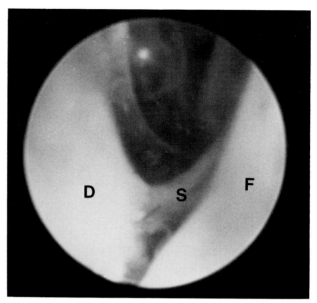

FIGURE 16–9. Arthroscopy of the canine left TMJ superior compartment. The view is more inferior than that shown in Figure 16–8 and demonstrates the inferior limit of the posterior recess. (D: disk; F: fossa; S: synovial reflection)

view to inspect this area. In this area a thin, synovial, lined anterior capsule can be found; its reflection onto the anterior margin of the fibrocartilaginous disk is also visible (Figs. 16–4, 16–5, 16–6, 16–7, 16–8, and 16–9).

SUMMARY

The canine model of TMJ arthroscopy has been used in investigative studies at our institution since 1986, specifically in experiments using fiberoptically guided neodymium-yttrium-aluminum-garnet (Nd:YAG) lasers within the TMJ. The model has additional potential for instructional applications, such as for use in orienting residents in the techniques of arthroscopy. If the crossbite distraction maneuver is accepted as a preliminary step in TMJ arthroscopy, then the convenience of the canine model can be exploited for investigative purposes (Table 16–2).

TABLE 16–2. ADVANTAGES AND DISADVANTAGES OF THE CANINE MODEL

Advantages	Disadvantages
Economical	Carnivore TMJ*
Easily anesthetized	Limited range of TMJ motion
Readily available	Anatomic discrepancies with
Institutionally friendly	respect to the human TMJ
Adequate size	Joint access requires more
Durable	maneuvering than with the
	human TMJ
	Variable local ethical
	acceptability

*Temporomandibular joint.

REFERENCES

1. Hilsabeck, RB; Laskin, DM. Arthroscopy of the temporomandibular joint of the rabbit. J Oral Surg (1978), 36:938–943.
2. Williams, RA; Laskin, DM. Arthroscopic examination of experimentally induced pathlogic conditions of the rabbit temporomandibular joint. J Oral Surg (1980), 38:652–659.
3. Holmlund, A; Hellsing, G; Bang, G. Arthroscopy of the rabbit temporomandibular joint. Int J Oral Maxillofac Surg (1986), 15:170–175.
4. Bosanquet, AG; Goss, AN. The sheep as a model for temporomandibular joint surgery. Int J Oral Maxillofac Surg (1987), 16:600–603.
5. Bosanquet, AG; Goss, AN. An animal model for TMJ arthroscopy. J Oral Maxillofac Surg (1989), 47:537–538.
6. Holmlund, A; Hellsing, G. Arthroscopy of the temporomandibular joint: An autopsy study. Int J Oral Surg (1985), 14:169–175.
7. Evans, HE; Christensen, GC. Miller's Anatomy of the Dog. 2nd Ed. Philadelphia: W.B. Saunders Company (1979), 229.

Seventeen

The Structure and Function of Sodium Hyaluronate and Its Use as a Biomaterial to Treat Temporomandibular Joint Dysfunction

DAVID A. SWANN, Ph.D.

Although the widespread use of hyaluronic acid (HA) products in medicine (commonly in the form of sodium hyaluronate) is a recent phenomenon, HA has been studied extensively since its discovery by Meyer in 1934.[1] It has been used as a biomaterial in the eye since the early 1960s, and patents concerned with the production of high-viscosity HA were filed in 1948 and 1949.[2,3]

The present period of HA use has been based on work carried out primarily at The Retina Foundation in Boston, Massachusetts. The initial studies used HA prepared from umbilical cord. The purpose of these studies was to develop a vitreous substitute to aid in the reattachment of the retina. This initial *artificial vitreous* was a composite of HA and collagen,[4,5] but HA alone later proved to be a more appropriate substance for this use.[6,7]

The use of HA to treat arthritic track horses has also been studied for quite a long time.[8] Whereas the early studies used human umbilical cord HA, the more recent use of rooster-comb HA was based on studies showing that HA can be purified from this tissue source in high yield by mild methods.[9] It had been shown previously by Boas[10] that rooster combs contained abundant quantities of HA, and physical and chemical studies by Laurent[11,12] had shown that rooster-comb HA has a high molecular weight similar to that of HAs isolated from umbilical cords. These experiments indicated that the rooster comb was the tissue of choice as a source of chemically pure, high-molecular-weight HA, that it could be isolated from this source by methods suitable for commercial production,[9,13] and that the purified HA was, therefore, considered an appropriate substance for use in humans.[14]

HA STRUCTURE AND ITS PROPERTIES

Chemical Structure

HA is defined as a linear polysaccharide composed of a repeating disaccharide unit [2-amino-2-deoxy-3-O-(B-D-glucopyranosyl uronic acid)-D-glucose] linked by 1-4β glycosidic bands (Fig. 17–1). This structure was established by enzymatic and chemical studies carried out on umbilical cord HA by Meyer[15] and was confirmed by chemical synthesis.[16] HAs isolated from

149

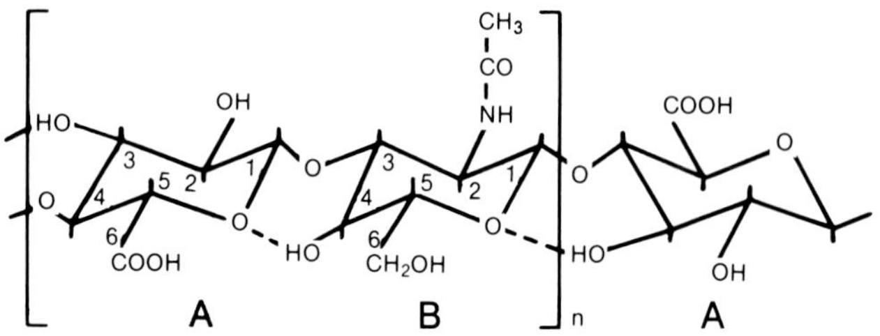

FIGURE 17–1. Chemical structure of sodium hyaluronate.

different tissues and from the capsules of bacteria have the same primary structure. Although the occurrence of other constituents in HA preparations has been reported, these have been shown to be either contaminants or analytic artifacts. The only differences between purified HAs from different sources are the length of the polysaccharide chains and their molecular weights.[17] The average molecular weight values reported in the literature range from a low of 70,000 for bovine vitreous HA[18] to 12×10^7 for a bovine synovial fluid HA.[19] Therefore, the value of n in Figure 17–1 can vary from 175 to 30,000. There is reason to believe, however, that some of the high values reported for the molecular weight of HA reflect the occurrence of aggregates or complexes involving interactions between HA polysaccharide chains[20–23] or HA and other constituents (Table 17–1).

Physical Properties

HA possesses a number of properties that make it useful as a biomaterial. Its high molecular weight, polyanionic structure, and large hydrodynamic molecular volume yield very viscous solutions at relatively low solute concentrations. These solutions act as non-Newtonian fluids[20] and also exhibit elasticity.[24] As a consequence, solutions of HA with a molecular weight of approximately 2×10^6 at a concentration of about 10 mg/ml act as a space-filling viscoelastic paste. The consistency can be altered by adjusting the molecular weight or the concentration of the solution, or both. HA polysaccharide chains in solution have a random coil configuration that possesses a certain degree of stiffness.[12,20,25] This stiffness is contributed by the polyanionic structure and the intramolecular hydrogen bonds[26,27] that limit movement at the glycosidic linkages.

X-ray studies have shown that HA polysaccharide chains can occur in different extended helical[28–31] and double-helical configurations.[32–34] It has also been shown that a water molecule can act as a bridge between adjacent carboxyl and N-acetyl groups and that the HA can assume two distinct stable conformations depending on the presence or the absence of this water-molecule bridge.[35] Circular dichroism studies

also support the occurrence of a double-stranded HA structure in the presence of organic solvents.[36]

Interactions with Other Macromolecules

The structure and the conformation of the polysaccharide chains allow HA to interact specifically with other macromolecules. The molecules that interact with HA are listed in Table 17–1.

Biologic Properties

Tissue Physiology. As a consequence of its chemical and physical structure and its interaction with other constituents, HA is thought to contribute to the functioning of tissues in several ways. It contributes to the osmotic pressure exerted by tissues.[51] HA molecules exclude other solute molecules from areas of solution,[52] thus increasing the effective concentration of the solute. The properties of systems in which HA is a component are very dependent on the HA concentration[51] and its molecular weight, but above certain concentrations (dependent on the molecular weight) HA occurs in solution as a network of chains, not as individual molecules.[53] Because of its occurrence as a network and its ability to exclude solutes, HA is able to influence a number of processes, such as the transport,[54,55] the reactivity, the conformation, and the solubility of solutes.

In addition, it appears that HA occurs in tissues in different forms. In synovial fluid it is present as a viscoelastic solution, whereas in cartilage and dermis it is normally present as a component of a complex, organized, extracellular matrix where it interacts specifically with other constituents (see Table 17–1). Swelling and induration in tissues may well result when trauma leads to the disruption of the indigenous structure of the extracellular matrix; when this occurs the HA becomes hydrodynamically effective, and fluid is trapped within the HA molecular domain.[56,57] As HA solutions exhibit a resistance to the bulk flow of water,[58]

TABLE 17–1. MOLECULAR INTERACTIONS INVOLVING HYALURONIC ACID

Constituent*	Reference Number(s) of Previous Research of Interaction
Proteoglycans	37, 38
Cartilage link proteins	39
Hyaluronectin	40
Fibronectin	41, 42
A novel protein	43
Cell surface receptors	44–48
Fibrinogen	49
Acute phase proteins	50

*Substances interacting with hyaluronic acid.

the swelling does not subside until the HA is removed from the tissue.

Tissue Lubrication. HA has been shown to act as a lubricant for soft tissues *in vitro*,[59,60] and it seems likely that HA performs this same function *in vivo* in joints, tendons, and ligaments.

In vitro studies have shown that the boundary lubricant for articular cartilage is a glycoprotein called lubricin,[61] but because HA is intimately associated with lubricin and other synovial fluid components it may contribute to cartilage lubrication in a synergistic manner, although this has not yet been demonstrated. The interactions between HA and articular cartilage glycoproteins and proteoglycans (see Table 17–1) also contribute to the integrity of articular cartilage and its function as a bearing surface.

Cell Migration in Development. Studies by Toole and coworkers[62,63] as well as other researchers[64,65] have shown that the synthesis of HA and its accumulation in extracellular matrices is associated with the migration of cells as part of developmental sequences of events.

HA has been shown to inhibit the differentiation of myoblasts.[66] However, HA has also been found to have a stimulatory effect on chondrogenesis that is dependent on the molecular weight of the HA.[67,68] This stimulatory effect was observed in the presence of HA with a molecular weight of $2-4 \times 10^5$; HA with a higher molecular weight (about 10^6) had no effect on this system.

Cell Invasion and Tumorigenesis. High concentrations of HA occur in the extracellular matrix of murine tumors. Concentrations have been shown to be especially high in peripheral zones of invasion in a rabbit V2 carcinoma.[69]

Tissue Repair. There appear to be parallels between the role of HA in developmental processes and its role in wound healing. HA is present in highest concentrations in the early stages of repair and is associated with fibroblast migration at the wound site.[70]

Angiogenesis. Studies have indicated that HA is able to promote angiogenesis.[71] A stimulatory effect was also observed in the presence of oligosaccharides that are produced by enzymatic degradation of HA.[72]

Inhibition of Proteoglycan Synthesis. HA has been shown to inhibit sulfate incorporation,[73] glycosaminoglycan synthesis,[74] and chondrocyte proteoglycan synthesis.[75]

Antigenicity. Early studies have shown that HA injected into animals and humans does not elicit an immunologic response.[76,77] More recent studies, however, have shown the presence of naturally occurring antibodies that cross react with HA.[78] It has also been shown that antibodies can be produced in mice if the appropriate antigen mixture is employed.[79,80]

Influence on Cell Behavior. A variety of phenomena that are dependent on the cell type and the test system employed have been reported. These phenomena are listed in Table 17–2.

HA SYNTHESIS

In eukaryotic cells, hyaluronate synthetase is an enzyme complex (450 kd) located in the plasma membrane.[101,102] HA synthesis in bacteria occurs because of the sequential addition of sugar moieties to the reducing end at the inside of the membrane. This is followed by extrusion of the HA polysaccharide chain to the exterior of the cell.[103–105]

Studies by Brecht and colleagues[98] indicate that there is a close relationship between HA synthesis and the sequence of events in the cell cycle. Cell rounding and detachment from the substratum is associated with increased HA synthesis. As the cells enter the S1 phase and resume spreading, HA synthesis drops sharply. Prehm and colleagues concluded that HA synthesis was a requirement for the completion of mitosis. HA synthesis is also associated with stimulated DNA synthesis.[108] HA synthesis is related to the growth phase of cells in culture,[109] and is suppressed by 5-bromode-

TABLE 17–2. THE EFFECTS OF HYALURONIC ACID (HA) ON CELL BEHAVIOR

Focus of Research	Reference Number(s) of Previous Research
Cell Movement	
In vivo association	
Migration of corneal mesenchymal cells	63
Migration of neural crest cells	64
Invasion of rabbit V2 carcinoma cells	67
In vitro enhancement	
Migration of cardiac cushion cells	81
Migration of chick embryo mesoderm cells	82
Migration of wound fibroblasts	83
Migration of choroid fibroblasts	84
Wound-healing granulation tissue cells	70
Migration of neutrophils	85
Inhibiting action	
Leukocyte locomotion	86, 87
Migration of neural crest cells	88
Migration of endothelial cells	71
Cell Adhesion	
Inhibition of neutrophil adhesion	89, 90
Cell Aggregation	
Inhibition of high HA concentration	89
Enhancement of low HA concentration	91–94
Via HA receptors	95, 96
Cell Proliferation	
Inhibition of high-molecular-weight HA	97
Fibroblast detachment and mitosis	98
Stimulation of lymphocyte proliferation due to mitogen inhibition	99
Leukocyte Functions	
Inhibition of phagocytosis at high HA concentration	87, 89
Stimulation of phagocytosis at low HA concentration	85, 100, 101

oxyuridine. However, HA synthesis was found to increase in proliferating cultures.[110] HA synthesis by synovial cells has been found to be increased by a monocyte cell factor,[111] and interleukin-1 has been observed to cause a ten-fold increase in fibroblast HA synthesis in culture.[112]

HA CATABOLISM

Studies conducted by Fraser and associates have shown that liver endothelial cells are able to bind circulating HA. Following endocytosis, the HA is catabolized into low-molecular-weight products.[113–116] A molecular weight of 25,000 was the upper limit for renally excreted HA.[113] More recent evidence indicates that the uptake of HA by the liver, the kidneys, and the spleen represents only a small part of the HA catabolized in the body and that the lymphatic system is the major site of HA uptake and breakdown.[117] In mammals hyaluronidases are endo β hexosaminidases[118] located in lysosomes;[151] and it is believed that HA is catabolized intracellularly following its uptake by mammalian cells. In addition, HA is degraded by free radicals generated by redox systems.[119] This process is catalyzed by heavy metals, such as copper and iron,[120] and may be of physiologic significance owing to the reaction between HA and ascorbate.[121,122]

THE MANUFACTURE OF MEDICAL-GRADE HA

MedChem Products, Inc. (Woburn, Massachusetts) was formed in 1970 to establish manufacturing methods for the production of HA that can be used as an implantable biomaterial to treat clinical disorders in humans and other animals. The proprietary methods established were based on published[9,13] as well as unpublished procedures.

Rooster combs are the basic tissue source used in both earlier and more recent production techniques. The combs are collected in a special manner. The HA is extracted and then subjected to a series of purification steps. The final sodium hyaluronate (NaHA) product is sterile, nonantigenic, nonpyrogenic, nontoxic, and noninflammatory. Depending on the use of the product, it can be formulated in different dosage forms. The types of NaHA products currently manufactured by MedChem are listed in Table 17–3.

CURRENT USES OF PRODUCTS CONTAINING HA

Ophthalmologic Applications

The success of HA as a biomaterial for use in ophthalmology is somewhat serendipitous in that it was

TABLE 17–3. HYALURONIC ACID (HA) PRODUCTS CURRENTLY AVAILABLE*

HA-containing Product	HA Concentration (mg/ml)	HA Molecular Weight	Clinical Uses
AMVISC	10–14	2×10^6	Intraocular surgical procedures
AMVISC Plus	14–18	$1–2 \times 10^6$	Intraocular surgical procedures
HYVISC	10–12	2×10^6	Intraarticular injection (in horses)
ORTHOVISC	10–16	2×10^6	Intraarticular injection (in the human temporomandibular joint)

*Products listed in this table are manufactured by MedChem Products, Inc.

designed as a vitreous substitute; however, HA only gained widespread use following the introduction of plastic intraocular lenses and as a result of the retrospective need for a device to aid in the surgical implantation of these lenses.[152]

Products such as AMVISC (see Table 17–3) that have been approved by the Food and Drug Administration (FDA) for ophthalmic use perform as viscoelastic surgical aids that lubricate and protect tissues by coating and maintaining spaces between adjacent tissue surfaces and by limiting the damage caused by devices and instruments. They are used primarily for the implantation of intraocular lenses and are regulated as Class III devices, which are subject to premarket approval. In addition to procedures for the extraction of a cataract and the implantation of an intraocular lens, AMVISC is also indicated for use in filtering surgery for glaucoma, procedures to reattach the retina, and corneal transplantation surgery.

The essential features of AMVISC that promote its use in ophthalmic surgical procedures are its biocompatibility (e.g., it is nontoxic, nonantigenic, nonpyrogenic, and noninflammatory) and its viscoelastic properties, which enable it to lubricate and separate cells and tissues and thereby protect them.

There is extensive literature on the intraocular use of HA that demonstrates both its safety and efficacy, with very few contraindications. Its space-maintaining and coating properties protect the cornea, reducing trauma to the iris.[123,124] The major problem associated with the use of HA in the implantation of intraocular lenses is a transient increase in intraocular pressure.[125]

In retina reattachment surgery[14] the viscoelastic HA acts as a tamponade, aiding in the repositioning of the retina and helping to maintain its realigned position following such procedures as cryothermy and diathermy.

Orthopedic Applications

Degenerative Joint Disease in Horses. The use of HA to treat joint disease in horses is a designed technique, which finds its basis in the occurrence of HA in synovial fluid and in the function of synovial fluid as a tissue lubricant. Preliminary studies in horses[8,126] indicate that intraarticular injections of HA are beneficial in the treatment of degenerative joint disease. Later studies[127–130] also demonstrated the safety and efficacy of HA use in horses. This beneficial effect of HA on joint function in these animals was demonstrated in controlled force plate studies.[131] The HA therapy was also more effective than conventional therapy in reducing the degree of lameness in horses with naturally occurring arthritic conditions[132] and in improving joint function in experimentally induced osteoarthritis.[133]

The use of HYVISC (see Table 17–3) is indicated in degenerative joint disease with associated synovitis. Following treatment with HYVISC, approximately 80% of horses show improvement in performance (training and track); however, as the effectiveness of this treatment persists long after the HA concentrations in the joint synovial fluid have returned to preinjection levels, the mechanism by which the improvement is attained is not clear.

Treatment of TMJ Dysfunction in Humans. The human ophthalmic and equine orthopedic uses of HA have satisfied most of the safety considerations regarding the use of this substance. Furthermore, a study in humans[134] has shown an improvement in clinical symptoms in osteoarthritic patients following the intraarticular injection of HA into the knee, the hip, and the elbow joints.

Based on this history of safety and on the potential usefulness of HA to treat human joint disease, we designed a study to evaluate the efficacy of HA for the treatment of TMJ disorders. Patients in the study were initially treated using normal, conservative procedures. Those patients who did not respond to conservative treatment and who would normally proceed to surgery were selected for ORTHOVISC treatment (see Table 17–3). This trial has indicated the efficacious properties of the product, and FDA approval for it is currently being sought.

Although few biochemical studies have been performed on temporomandibular joint (TMJ) synovial fluid, it appears that lubricating mechanisms in the TMJ and other joints are similar in both bovines and humans.[135] The efficacy of exogenous HA in improving joint function is believed to be based upon a number of factors. Probably the most important is the ability of HA to act as a hydrodynamic lubricant.[59,60] When it is used, frictional interactions between tissue surfaces are decreased, resulting in a decrease in irritation and mechanical trauma. In the equine studies, however, a long-term response was observed following intraarticular injection. This response extended beyond the expected residence time for HA in the injected joint. This indicated that HA may be selectively retained by joint cells or may have an effect on them, accounting for this phenomenon. The possible effects of HA on cell behavior are presented in Table 17–2.

Studies carried out in rabbits have shown that repeated HA injections are well tolerated[136] but had no effect on the healing of cartilaginous or osteochondral lesions.[137] This may indicate that such lesions are not contributing factors; however, HA may exert an effect by virtue of its influence on chondrocytes[73,74] and via its interactions with cartilage-matrix glycoproteins[39] and proteoglycans.[37,38] It has been shown in rabbits[138] that labeled HA injected into the knee joint can penetrate articular cartilage. Exogenous HA injections may also improve joint function by affecting immune and inflammatory processes (see Table 17–2), or by influencing the duration of actions and responses to endogenous bioactive agents in a manner similar to that demonstrated for anesthetic agents and pilocarpine.[139–142]

An additional beneficial effect related to the lubricating properties of HA and its effect on cell behavior is the evidence that HA can aid in the prevention of adhesion formation. One early study[143] has shown the occurrence of a decreased fibrotic response following the injection of HA at wound sites. More recent experiments have indicated that HA reduces tension[144,145] and peritoneal adhesions,[146] and may be useful after jejunoileal bypass surgery.[147] HA decreases scar formation following joint immobilization,[148] laminectomy,[149] and strabismus surgery.[150]

REFERENCES

1. Meyer, K; Palmer, J. Polysaccharide of vitreous humor. J Biol Chem (1934) 107:629–634.
2. Hadidian, Z; Pirie, M. Process for the production of high-viscosity hyaluronic acid. U.S. Patent #2,583,096. Assignee: GD Searle & Co., Chicago.
3. Hadidian, Z; Pirie, M. Production of high viscosity hyaluronic acid. U.S. Patent #2,585,546. Assignee: GD Searle & Co., Skokie, Illinois.
4. Sweeney, DB; Balazs, EA. Fate of collagen and hyaluronic acid gels and solutions injected in vitreous of the owl monkey. Invest Ophthalmol Vis Sci (1964), 3:473.
5. Balazs, FA; Sweeney, DB. The use of hyaluronic acid and collagen preparation in eye surgery. *In:* Schepens, CL; Regan, CDJ, eds. Controversial Aspects of the Management of Retinal Detachment. Boston: Little, Brown & Co. (1965), 200.
6. Hruby, K. Further experiences with hyaluronic acid as replacement of the vitreous body in retinal detachment. Bibl Ophthalmol (1966), 70:228.
7. Balazs, EA; Hultsch, E. Replacement of the vitreous with hyaluronic acid, collagen and other polymers. *In:* Irvine, AR; O'Malley, C, eds. Advances in Vitreous Surgery. Springfield, Illinois: Charles C Thomas (1976), 601–625.

8. Rydell, NH; Butler, J; Balazs, EA. Hyaluronic acid in synovial fluid: II. Effect of intraarticular injection of hyaluronic acid on the clinical symptoms of arthritis in track horses. Acta Vet Scand (1970), 11:139–155.

9. Swann, DA. Studies on hyaluronic acid: I. The preparation and properties of rooster comb hyaluronic acid. Biochim Biophys Acta (1968), 156:17–30.

10. Boas, N. Isolation of hyaluronic acid from the cock's comb. J Biol Chem (1949), 181:573–575.

11. Laurent, TC. A comparative study of physico-chemical properties of hyaluronic acid prepared according to different methods and from different tissues. Arkiv für Kemi (1955), 11:487–496.

12. Laurent, TC; Gergely, J. Light scattering studies on hyaluronic acid. J Biol Chem (1955), 212:325–333.

13. Swann, DA. Studies on hyaluronic acid: II. The protein component(s) of rooster comb hyaluronic acid. Biochim Biophys Acta (1968b) 160:96–105.

14. Pruett, RC; Schepens, CL; Swann, DA. Hyaluronic acid vitreous substitute: A six-year clinical evaluation. Arch Ophthalmol (1979), 97:2325.

15. Meyer, K. Chemical structure of hyaluronic acid. Fed Proc (1958), 17:1075.

16. Jeanloz, RW; Jeanloz; DA. The degradation of hyaluronic acid by methanolysis. Biochemistry (1964), 3:121.

17. Laurent, TC. In: Balazs, EA, ed. Chemistry and Molecular Biology of the Intracellular Matrix. Vol. II. New York: Academic Press (1970), 703–732.

18. Varga, L. Studies on hyaluronic acid prepared from the vitreous body. J Biol Chem (1955), 217:651.

19. Silpananta, P; Dunstone, JR; Ogston, AG. Fractionation of a hyaluronic acid preparation in a density gradient: Some properties of the hyaluronic acid. Biochem J (1968), 109:43–50.

20. Ogston, AG; Stanier, JE. The dimensions of the particle of hyaluronic acid complex in synovial fluid. Biochem J (1951), 49:585.

21. Welsh, EJ; Rees, DA; Morris, ER; Madden, JK. Competitive inhibition evidence for specific intermolecular interactions in hyaluronate solutions. J Mol Biol (1980), 138:375–382.

22. Silver, FH; Swann, DA. Laser light scattering measurements on vitreous and rooster comb hyaluronate acids. Int J Macromol (1982), 4:425–429.

23. Turner, RE; Lin, PY; Cowman, MK. Self-association of hyaluronate segments in aqueous NaCl solution. Arch Biochem Biophys (1988), 265:484–495.

24. Ogston, AG; Stanier, JE. Discuss Faraday Soc (1953), 13:275.

25. Laurent, TC; Ryan, M; Pietruszkiewicz, A. Fractionation of hyaluronic acid: The polydispersity of hyaluronic acid from the bovine vitreous body. Biochim Biophys Acta (1960), 42:476–485.

26. Atkins, EDT; Meader, D; Scott, JE. Model for hyaluronic acid incorporating four intramolecular hydrogen bonds. Int J Biol Macromol (1980), 2:318–319.

27. Scott, JE; Heatley, F; Hull, WD. Secondary structure of hyaluronate in solution: A 1H-n.m.r. investigation at 300 and 500 MHz in [2H6] dimethyl sulphoxide solution. Biochem J (1984), 220:197–205.

28. Atkins, EDT; Sheehan, JK. Hyaluronates: Relation between molecular conformations. Science (1973), 179:562.

29. Sheehan, J; Atkins, E; Nieduszynski, I. Studies on the connective tissue polysaccharides: Two-dimensional packing schemes for three-fold hyaluronate chains. J Mol Biol (1975), 91:153.

30. Winter, WT; Smith, PJC; Arnott, S. Hyaluronic acid: Structure of a fully extended 3-fold helical sodium salt and comparison with the less extended 4-fold helical forms. J Mol Biol (1975), 99:219–235.

31. Winter, WT; Arnott, S. Hyaluronic acid: The role of divalent cations in conformation and packing. J Mol Biol (1977), 177:761–784.

32. Dea, ICM; Moorhouse, R; Rees, DA; et al. Hyaluronic acid: A novel, double-helical molecule. Science (1973), 179:560–562.

33. Sheehan, JK; Gardner, KH; Atkins, EDT. Hyaluronic acid: A double-helical structure in the presence of potassium at low pH and found also with the cations ammonium, rubidium and caesium. J Mol Biol (1977), 117:113–135.

34. Arnott, S; Mitra, AK; Raghunathan, S. Hyaluronic acid double helix. J Mol Biol (1983), 169:861–872.

35. Heatley, F; Scott, JE. A water molecule participates in the secondary structure of hyaluronan. Biochem J (1988), 254:489–493.

36. Staskus, PW; Johnson, WC. Double-stranded structure for hyaluronic acid in ethanol-aqueous solution as revealed by circular dichroism of oligomers. Biochemistry (1988), 27:1528–1534.

37. Hardingham, T; Muir, H. The specific interaction of hyaluronic acid with cartilage proteoglycans. Biochim Biophys Acta (1972), 279:401–405.

38. Hardingham, TE; Muir, H. Binding of oligosaccharides of hyaluronic acid to proteoglycans. Biochem J (1973), 135:905–908.

39. Tengblad, A. A comparative study of the binding of cartilage link protein and the hyaluronate-binding region of the cartilage proteoglycan to hyaluronate-substituted Sepharose gel. Biochem J (1981), 199:297–305.

40. Delpech, B; Halavent, C. Characterization and purification from human brain of a hyaluronic acid–binding glycoprotein, hyaluronectin. J Neurochem (1981), 36:855–859.

41. Yamada, KM; Kennedy, DW; Kimata, K; Pratt, RM. Characterization of fibronectin interactions with glycosaminoglycans and identification of active proteolytic fragments. J Biol Chem (1980), 255:6055–6063.

42. Isemura, M: Yosizawa, Z; Koide, T; Ono, T. Interaction of fibronectin and its proteolytic fragments with hyaluronic acid. J Biochem (Tokyo) (1982), 91:731–734.

43. D'Souza, M; Datta, K. A novel protein that binds to hyaluronic acid. Biochem Int (1986), 13:79–88.

44. Underhill, CB; Toole, BP. Physical characteristics of hyaluronate binding to the surface of simian virus 40–transformed 3T3 cells. J Biol Chem (1980), 255:4544–4549.

45. Turley, EA; Torrance, J. Localization of hyaluronate and hyaluronate-binding protein on motile and non-motile fibroblasts. Exp Cell Res (1984), 161:17–28.

46. Underhill, CB; Thurn, AL; Lacey, BE. Characterization and identification of the hyaluronate-binding site from membranes of SV-3T3 cells. J Biol Chem (1985), 260:8128–8133.

47. Laurent, TC; Fraser, JRE; Pertoft, H; Sedsrod, B. Binding of hyaluronate and chondroitin sulphate to liver endothelial cells. Biochem J (1986), 234:653–658.

48. Green, SJ; Tarone, G; Underhill, CB. Distribution of hyaluronate and hyaluronate receptors in the adult lung. J Cell Sci (1988), (Part I):145–156.

49. LeBoeuf, RD; Raja, RH; Fuller, GM; Weigel, PH. Human fibrinogen specifically binds hyaluronic acid. J Biol Chem (1986), 261:12586–12592.

50. Chang, NS; Boackle, RJ; Armand, G. Hyaluronic acid–complement interactions: I. Reversible heat-induced anticomplementary activity. Mol Immunol (1985), 22:391–397.

51. Laurent, TC; Ogston, AG. The interaction between polysaccharides and other macromolecules: The osmotic pressure of mixtures of serum albumin and hyaluronic acid. Biochem J (1963), 89:249–253.

52. Ogston, AG; Phelps, CF. The partition of solutes between buffer solutions and solutions containing hyaluronic acid. Biochem J (1960), 78:827–833.

53. Ogston, AG; Keaton, BN; Wells, JD. On the transport of compact particles through solutions of chain polymers. Proc Roy Soc Lond A (1973), 333:297–309.

54. Laurent, TC; Bjork, I; Pietruskiewicz, A; Persson, H. On the interaction between polysaccharides and other macromolecules: II Transport of globular particles through hyaluronic acid. Biochim Biophys Acta (1963), 78:351–359.

55. Preston, BN; Laurent, TC; Comper, WD; Checkley, GJ. Rapid polymer transport in concentrated solutions through the formation of ordered structures. Nature (1980), 287:499–503.

56. Klein, J; Meyer, FA. Tissue structure and macromolecular diffusion in umbilical cord: Immobilization of endogenous hyaluronic acid. Biochim Biophys Acta (1983), 755:400–411.

57. Meyer, FA. Macromolecular basis of globular protein exclusion and of swelling pressure in loose connective tissue (umbilical cord). Biochim Biophys Acta (1983), 755:388–399.

58. Jackson, GW; James, DF. The hydrodynamic resistance of

hyaluronic acid and its contribution to tissue permeability. Biorheology (1982), 19:317–330.

59. Radin, EL; Paul, IL; Swann, DA; Schottstaedt, ES. Lubrication of synovial membrane. Ann Rheum Dis (1971), 30:322–325.

60. Swann, DA; Radin, EL; Nazimiec, M; et al. Role of hyaluronic acid in joint lubrication. Ann Rheum Dis (1974), 33:318–326.

61. Swann, DA; Slayter, HS; Silver, FH. The molecular structure of lubricating glycoprotein-I, the boundary lubricant for articular cartilage. J Biol Chem (1981), 256:5921–5925.

62. Toole, BP; Gross, J. The extracellular matrix of the regenerating newt limb: Synthesis and removal of hyaluronate prior to differentiation. Dev Biol (1971), 25:57–77.

63. Toole, BP; Trelstad, RL. Hyaluronate production and removal during corneal development in the chick. Dev Biol (1971), 26:28–35.

64. Pratt, RM; Larsen, MA; Johnston, MC. Migration of cranial neural crest cells in a cell-free hyaluronate-rich matrix. Dev Biol (1975), 44:298–305.

65. Markwald, RR; Fitzharris, TP; Bank, H; Bernanke, DH. Structural analysis of the matrical organization of glycosaminoglycans. Dev Biol (1978), 62:292–316.

66. Kujawa, MJ; Pechak, DJ; Fizman, MY; Caplan, AI. Hyaluronic acid bonded to cell culture surfaces inhibits the program of myogenesis. Dev Biol (1986), 133:10–16.

67. Kujawa, MJ; Carrino, DA; Caplan, AI. Substrate-bonded hyaluronic acid exhibits a size-dependent stimulation of chondrogenic differentiation of stage 24 limb mesenchymal cells in culture. Dev Biol (1986), 114:519–528.

68. Kujawa, MJ; Caplan, AI. Hyaluronic acid bonded to cell culture and substrate surfaces stimulates chondrogenesis in stage 24 limb mesenchyme cell cultures. Dev Biol (1986), 114:504–518.

69. Toole, BP; Biswas, C; Gross, J. Hyaluronate and invasiveness of the rabbit V2 carcinoma. Proc Natl Acad Sci U S A (1979), 76:6299–6303.

70. Abatangelo, G; Martelli, M; Vecchia, P. Healing of hyaluronic acid–enriched wounds: Histological observations. J Surg Res (1983), 35:410–416.

71. Feinberg, RN; Beebe, DC. Hyaluronate in vasculogenesis. Science (1983), 220:1177–1179.

72. West, DC; Hampson, IN; Arnold, F; Kumar, S. Angiogenesis induced by degradation products of hyaluronate. Science (1985), 228:1324–1326.

73. Wiebkin, OW; Muir, H. The inhibition of sulphate incorporation in isolated adult chondrocytes by hyaluronic acid. FEBS Lett (1973), 37:42–46.

74. Solursh, M; Vacreivyck, SA; Rorter, RC. Depression by HA of GAG synthesis by cultured chick embryo chondrocytes. Dev Biol (1974), 41:233–244.

75. Bansal, MK; Ward, H; Mason, RM. Proteoglycan synthesis in suspension cultures of Swarm rat chondrosarcoma chondrocytes and inhibition by exogenous hyaluronate. Arch Biochem Biophys (1986), 246:602–610.

76. Richter, W. Non-immunogenicity of purified hyaluronic acid preparations tested by passive cutaneous anaphylaxis. Arch Allergy (1974), 47:211–217.

77. Richter, AW; Ryde, EM; Zetterstrom, EO. Non-immunologenicity of a purified sodium hyaluronate preparation in man. Int Arch Allergy Appl Immunol (1979), 59:45–48.

78. Underhill, CB. Naturally-occurring antibodies which bind hyaluronate. Biochem Biophys Res Commun (1982), 108:129–130.

79. Fillit, HM; McCarty, M; Blake, M. Induction of antibodies to hyaluronic acid by immunization of rabbits with encapsulated streptococci. J Exp Med (1986), 164:762–776.

80. Fillit, HM; Blake, M; MacDonald, C; McCarthy, M. Immunogenicity of liposome-bound hyaluronate in mice: At least two different antigenic sites on hyaluronate are identified by mouse monoclonal antibodies. J Exp Med (1988), 168:971–982.

81. Bernanke, DH; Markwold, RR. Effects of two glycosaminoglycans on seeding of cardiac cushion cells into a collagen lattice culture system. Anat Rec (1984), 210:25–31.

82. Sanders, EJ; Prasad, S. The culture of chick embryo mesoderm cells in hydrated collagen gels. J Exp Zool (1983), 226:81–92.

83. Doillon, CJ; Silver, FH. Collagen-based wound dressing: Effects of hyaluronic acid and fibronectin on wound healing. Biomaterials (1986), 7:3–8.

84. Docherty, R: Forrester, JV; Lackies, JM; Gregory, DW. Glycosaminoglycans facilitate the movement of fibroblasts through three-dimensional collagen matrices. J Cell Sci (1989), 72:263–270.

85. Hakansson, L; Venge, P. The molecular basis of the hyaluronic acid–mediated stimulation of granulocyte function. J Immunol (1987), 138:4347–4352.

86. Balazs, EA; Darzynkiewicz, Z. The effect of hyaluronic acid on fibroblasts, mononuclear phagocytes and lymphocytes. In: Kulonen, E; Pikkarainen, J, eds. Biology of the Fibroblast. I. London: Academic Press (1973), 237.

87. Forrester, JV; Wilkinson, PC. Inhibition of leukocyte locomotion by hyaluronic acid. J Cell Sci (1981), 48:315–331.

88. Turley, EA; Bowman, P; Kytryk, MA. Effects of hyaluronate and hyaluronate-binding proteins on cell motile and contact behavior. J Cell Sci (1985), 78:133–145.

89. Forrester, JV; Lackie, JM. Effect of hyaluronic acid on neutrophil adhesion. J Cell Sci (1981), 50:329–344.

90. Abatangelo, G; Cortivo, R; Martelli, M; Vecchia, P. Cell detachment mediated by hyaluronic acid. Exp Cell Res (1982), 137:73–78.

91. Pessac, B; Defendi, V. Cell aggregation: Role of acid mucopolysaccharides. Science (1972), 175:898–900.

92. Wasteson, A; Wetermark, B; Lindahl, U; Ponten, J. Aggregation of feline lymphoma cells by hyaluronic acid. Int J Cancer (1973), 12:169–178.

93. Wright, TC; Underhill, CB; Toole, BP; Karnovsky, MJ. Divalent cation-independent aggregation of rat fibroblasts infected with a temperature-sensitive mutant of Rous sarcoma virus. Cancer Res (1981), 41:5107–5113.

94. Green, SJ; Tarone, G; Underhill, CB. Aggregation of macrophages and fibroblasts is inhibited by a monoclonal antibody to the hyaluronate receptor. Exp Cell Res (1988), 178:224–232.

95. Underhill, CB; Toole, BP. Receptors for hyaluronate on the surface of parent and virus-transformed cell lines: Binding and aggregation studies. Exp Cell Res (1981), 131:419–423.

96. Underhill, CB. Interaction of hyaluronate with the surface of Simian virus 40–transformed 3T3 cells: Aggregation and binding studies. J Cell Sci (1982), 56:177–189.

97. Goldberg, RL; Toole, BP. Hyaluronate inhibition of cell proliferation. Arthritis Rheum (1987), 30:769–778.

98. Brecht, M; Mayer, U; Schlosser, E; Prehm, P. Increased hyaluronate synthesis is required for fibroblast detachment and mitosis. Biochem J (1986), 239:445–450.

99. Darzynkiewicz, Z; Balazs, EA. Effect of connective tissue intercellular matrix on lymphocyte stimulation: I. Suppression of lymphocyte stimulation by hyaluronic acid. Exp Cell Res (1971), 66:113–123.

100. Hakansson, L; Hallgren, R; Venge, P; et al. Hyaluronic acid stimulates neutrophil function in vitro and in vivo: A review of experimental results and a presentation of a preliminary clinical trial. Scand J Infect Dis Suppl (1980), 24:54–57.

101. Mian, N. Analysis of cell growth phase-related variations in hyaluronate synthase activity of isolated plasma-membrane fractions of cultured human skin fibroblasts. Biochem J (1986), 237:333–342.

102. Mian, N. Character of a high-Mr plasma-membrane-bound protein and assessment of its role as a constituent of hyaluronate synthase complex. Biochem J (1986), 237:343–357.

103. Prehm, P. Synthesis of hyaluronate in differentiated teratocarcinoma cells: Characterization of the synthase. Biochem J (1983), 211:181–189.

104. Prehm, P. Synthesis of hyaluronate in differentiated teratocarcinoma cells: Mechanism of chain growth. Biochem J (1983), 21:191–198.

105. Prehm, P. Hyaluronate is synthesized at plasma membranes. Biochem J (1984), 220:597–600.

106. Cohn, RH; Cassiman, JJ; Bernfield, MR. Relationship of transformation, all density and growth control to the cellular distribution of newly synthesized GAG. J Cell Biol (1976), 71:280–294.

107. Hronowski, L; Anastassiades, TP. The effect of cell density on net rates of GAG synthesis and secretion by cultured rat fibroblasts. J Biol Chem (1980), 255:10091–10099.

108. Moscatelli, D; Rubin, H. Increased HA production on stimulation of DNA synthesis in chick embryo fibroblasts. Nature (1975), 254:65–66.

109. Tomida, M; Koyama, H; Ono, R. Hyaluronic acid synthetase in cultured mammalian cells producing hyaluronic acid: Oscillatory change during growth phase and suppression with 5-bromodeoxyuridine. Biochim Biophys Acta (1974), 338:352–363.

110. Tomida, M; Koyama, H; Ono, R. Induction of hyaluronic acid synthesis activity in rat fibroblasts by media change of confluent cultures. J Cell Physiol (1975), 86:121–130.

111. Bocquet, J; Langris, M; Daireaux, M; et al. Mononuclear cell-mediated modulation of synovial cell metabolism: II. Increased hyaluronic acid synthesis by a monocyte cell factor (MCF). Exp Cell Res (1985), 160:9–18.

112. Bronson, RE; Bertolami, CN; Siebert, EP. Modulation of fibroblast growth and glycosaminoglycan synthesis by interleukin-1. Coll Rel Res (1987), 7:323–332.

113. Fraser, JR; Laurent, TC; Pertoft, H; Baxter, E. Plasma clearance, tissue distribution and metabolism of hyaluronic acid injected intravenously in the rabbit. Biochem J (1981), 200:415–424.

114. Fraser, JR; Appelgren, LE; Laurent, TC. Tissue uptake of circulating hyaluronic acid. A whole body autoradiographic study. Cell Tissue Res (1983), 233:285–293.

115. Fraser, JRE; Laurent, TC; Engström-Laurent, A; Laurent, UBG. Elimination of hyaluronic acid from the bloodstream in the human. Clin Exp Pharmacol Physiol (1984), 11:17–25.

116. Fraser, JR; Alcorn, D; Laurent, TC; et al. Uptake of circulating hyaluronic acid by the rat liver: Cellular localization in situ. Cell Tissue Res (1985), 242:505–510.

117. Fraser, JR; Kimpton, WG; Laurent, TC; Cahill, RN; Vakakis, N. Uptake and degradation of hyaluronan in lymphatic tissue. Biochem J (1988), 256:153–158.

118. Gibian, H. Hyaluronidases in the Amino Sugars. Jeanloz, R; Balazs, EA, eds. New York: Academic Press (1968).

119. Sunblad, L; Balazs, EA. Chemical and physical changes of glycosaminoglycans and glycoproteins caused by oxidation-reduction systems and radiation. In Balazs, EA; Jeanloz, RW, eds. The Amino Sugars. Vol. IIB. New York: Academic Press (1968), 229–250.

120. Wong, SF; Halliwell, B; Richmond, R; Skowroneck, WR. The role of superoxide and hydroxyl radicals in the degradation of hyaluronic acid induced by metal ions and by ascorbic acid. J Inorg Biochem (1981), 14:127–134.

121. Swann, DA. Studies on the structure of hyaluronic acid: Characterization of product formed when hyaluronic acid is treated with ascorbic acid. Biochem J (1969), 114:819–825.

122. Cleland, RL; Stoolmiller, AC; Roden, L; Laurent, TC. Partial characterization of reaction products formed by the degradation of hyaluronic acid with ascorbic acid. Biochim Biophys Acta (1969), 192:385–394.

123. Miller, D; O'Connor, P; Williams, J. HA reduced corneal thickness and trauma to iris. Use of Na-hyaluronate during intraocular lens implantation in rabbits. Ophthalmic Surg (1977), 8:58–61.

124. Miller, D; Stegmann, R. Use of Na-hyaluronate in anterior segment eye surgery. J Am Intraocul Implant Soc (1980), 6:13–15.

125. MacRae, SM; Edelhauser, HF; Hyrdiule, RA; et al. The effects of sodium hyaluronate, chondroitin sulfate, and methylcellulose on the corneal endothelium and intraocular pressure. Am J Ophthalmol (1983), 95:332–341.

126. Rydell, N; Balazs, EA. Effect of intra-articular injection of hyaluronic acid on the clinical symptoms of osteoarthritis and on granulation tissue formation. Clin Orthop (1971), 80:25–32.

127. Asheim, A; Lindblad, G. Intra-articular treatment of arthritis in race-horses with sodium hyaluronate. Acta Vet Scand (1976), 17:379–394.

128. Rose, RJ. The intra-articular use of sodium hyaluronate for the treatment of osteoarthrosis in the horse. N Z Vet J (1979), 27:5–8.

129. Irwin, DH. Sodium hyaluronate in equine traumatic arthritis. J S Afr Vet Assoc (1980), 51:231–233.

130. Auer, JA; Fackelman, GE, Gingerich, DA; Fetter, AW. Effect of hyaluronic acid in naturally occurring and experimentally induced osteoarthritis. Am J Vet Res (1980), 41:568–574.

131. Gingerich, DA; Auer, JA; Fackelman, GE. Force plate studies on the effect of exogenous hyaluronic acid on joint function in equine arthritis. J Vet Pharmcol Ther (1979), 2:291–298.

132. Ruth, DT; Swites, BJ. Comparison of the effectiveness of intra-articular hyaluronic acid and conventional therapy for the treatment of naturally occurring arthritic conditions in horses. Vet Clin North Am Equine Pract (1985), 7:25–29.

133. Gingerich, DA; Auer, JA; Fackelman, GE. Effect of exogenous hyaluronic acid on joint function in experimentally induced equine osteoarthritis: Dosage titration studies. Res Vet Sci (1981), 30:192–197.

134. Peyron, JG; Balazs, EA. Preliminary clinical assessment of sodium hyaluronate injection into human arthritic joints. Path Biol (1974), 22:731.

135. Hatton, MN; Swann, DA. Studies on bovine temporomandibular joint synovial fluid. J Prosthet Dent (1986), 56:635–638.

136. Wigren, A; Wik, O; Falk, J. Intra-articular injection of HMW HA: An experimental study on normal adult rabbit knee joints to study the effect of repeated HA injections over a period of 8 weeks. Acta Orthop Scand (1976), 47:480–485.

137. Wigren, A; Falk, J; Wik, O. The healing of cartilage injuries under the influence of joint immobilization and repeated HA injections. Acta Orthop Scand (1978), 49:121–133.

138. Antonas, KN; Fraser, JRE; Muirden, KD. Distribution of biologically labelled radioactive hyaluronic acid injected into joints. Ann Rheum Dis (1973), 32:103–111.

139. Hassan, HG; Akerman, B; Renck, H; et al. Effects of adjuvants to local anaesthetics on their duration: III. Experimental studies of hyaluronic acid. Acta Anaesthesiol Scand (1985), 29:384–388.

140. Johansson, A; Hassan, H; Renck, H. Effects of adjuvants to local anaesthetics on their duration: IV. Effect of hyaluronic acid added to bupivacaine or prilocaine on the duration of nerve blockade in man. Acta Anaesthesiol Scand (1985), 29:736–738.

141. Renck, H; Hassan, HG; Lindberg, B; Akerman, B. Effects of macromolecular adjuvants on the duration of prilocaine: Experimental studies on the effect of variations of viscosity and sodium content and of inclusion of adrenaline. Acta Anaesthesiol Scand (1988), 32:355–364.

142. Camber, O; Edman, P; Guerney, R. Influence of sodium hyaluronate on the meiotic effect of pilocarpine in rabbits. Curr Eye Res (1987), 6:779–784.

143. Rydell, N. Decreased granulation tissue reaction after installment of HA. Acta Orthop Scand (1970), 41:307–311.

144. St. Onge, R; Weiss, C; Denlinger, JL; Balazs, EA. A preliminary assessment of Na-hyaluronate injection into "no man's land" for primary flexor tendon repair. Clin Orthop (1980), 146:269–275.

145. Thomas, SC; Jones, LC; Hungerford, DS. Hyaluronic acid and its effect of postoperative adhesions in the rabbit flexor tendon: A preliminary look. Clin Orthop (1986), 206:281–289.

146. Bergqvist, D; Arfors, KE. Effect of dextran and hyaluronic acid on the development of postoperative peritoneal adhesions in experimental animals. Eur Surg Res (1979), 9:321–325.

147. Trabucchi, E; Foschi, D; Marazzi, M; et al. Prevention of wound dehiscence in severely obese patients with jejuno-ileal bypass: The role of hyaluronic acid. Pharmatherapeutica (1988), 5:233–239.

148. Amiel, D; Frey, C; Woo, SL; et al. Value of hyaluronic acid in the prevention of contracture formation. Clin Orthop (1985), 196:306–311.

149. Weiss, C; Dennis, J; Suros, JM; et al. Sodium hylan for the prevention of postlaminectomy scar formation. Orth Res Society, Las Vegas (1989), 14:44.

150. Searl, SS; Metz, HS; Lindahl, KJ. The use of sodium hyaluronate as a biologic sleeve in strabismus surgery. Ann Ophthalmol (1987), 19:259–262.

151. Aronson, NN; Davidson, EA. Lysosomal hyaluronidase from rat liver. I. Preparation. J Biol Chem (1967), 242:437, 441.

152. Miller, D; Stegmann, R. Use of Na-hyaluronate in anterior segment eye surgery. Am Intraocular Implant Soc (1980), 6:13.

Eighteen

Sodium Hyaluronate Injections in Synovial Joints

CHANGRUI LIU, D.D.S.
GLENN T. CLARK, D.D.S., M.S.

Hyaluronic acid (HA), a naturally occurring polysaccharide, was first discovered in 1934 in the vitreous fluid of the eye, and later in synovial fluid, umbilical cord, rooster combs, and in lesser amounts, in the extracellular matrix of connective tissue throughout the body.[1–3] Based on its biologic and physical properties, HA is considered to be an important tissue lubricant.[4,5] It has also been proposed that synovial fluid, which contains high concentrations of HA, acts as a nutrient source for the avascular articular cartilage cells and synovial membrane.[6]

THE RESEARCH BASIS FOR THE ROLE OF SODIUM HYALURONATE IN SYNOVIAL JOINTS

HA, in the form of its sodium salt sodium hyaluronate, was first used clinically to protect tissues during ophthalmic surgery.[7] Even prior to its ophthalmic use, HA was proposed as a therapeutic agent for synovial joint surfaces owing to its lubricating and shock-absorbing properties.[6,8–10] This section of the chapter concentrates on the research underlying clinical applications of HA in both human and animal joint diseases.

Lubrication Function of Hyaluronate

The therapeutic potential of HA is substantiated on the basic biochemical and physical chemistry studies that have characterized its structure and function. Linear HA chains in solution intertwine and form a complex three-dimensional network of molecules, thus providing HA with its lubricating and shock-absorbing properties.[11] Solutions of HA are also very viscous and therefore considerably resistant to flow.[12] This resistance is partially responsible for HA's tendency to stay within the joint capsule. The limited space between the polysaccharide chains of HA's complex three-dimensional form acts to exclude other macromolecular solutes from the compartment it occupies. In other words, the more tightly woven the three-dimensional network and the larger the size of the solute molecule, the more other solutes will be excluded.[11,13–15]

HA may also bind or be adsorbed onto the thin (1–2 μm), protein-containing, amorphous surface layer of the articular cartilage, and this action undoubtedly contributes to lubrication.[8,16–18] Data clearly suggest that the protective function of this coating is vital to joint health.

Synovectomy has been shown to cause this amorphous layer to disappear, resulting in degenerative changes of the cartilage. The role of HA in the formation of this coating was demonstrated when an intraarticular injection was found to inhibit the disappearance of this layer in synovectomized rabbit knee joints.[19] These data also support the theory that HA plays an important role in maintaining normal cartilage surface and in protecting the synovial membrane.[20]

The probable mechanism by which HA provides this protection is its ability to bind or become adsorbed to the articular cartilage surface, forming an elastic cushion between joint surfaces.[19,20] The protection conferred by HA is thought to be better under dynamic conditions owing to HA solutions' viscoelastic properties.[21,22] In addition, an HA-rich amorphous coating probably functions to prevent cartilage degradation by acting as a barrier to the invasion of various catabolic enzymes into the articular cartilage.[23] Chondrocyte activity inhibition, as well as decreased transformation and stimulation of lymphocytes, has been shown to be influenced by HA.[18,24,25]

Synovial Joint Disease and HA

The pathologic effects of arthritis and arthrosis (chronic or acute) on synovial fluid and joint surfaces in human and equine joints have been described.[26] These effects include decreased elasticity of the joint surfaces and reduced viscosity of the synovial fluid. There is also a reduction in the size of individual HA molecules as well as a much lower concentration of HA found in the joint fluid of a typical arthritic patient.[8,10,27,28] Osteoarthritis has been shown to reduce the aggregation of the proteoglycan macromolecular complexes on exposed joint cartilage.[29-32] Also, the average molecular weight of HA is reduced in rheumatoid arthritis.[10,33]

It has also been observed that the viscosity and elasticity of synovial fluid is reduced in acutely inflamed human joints.[28,34] A study conducted by Peyron and Balazs in 1974 determined the average limiting viscosity of the knee, the hip, and the elbow joints to be 2400 ml/g in untreated arthritis patients. (The normal human knee synovial fluid limiting viscosity has an average value of 5200 ml/g.) After multiple injections of HA the average limiting viscosity was 3600 ml/g.[35]

Other research has shown that the synovial fluid of rheumatoid arthritis patients does not show high mucin clot formation and that an increase in the rate of mucin formation occurs after an injection of HA.[20,36] Overall, these data support the hypothesis that HA plays an important role in maintaining normal synovial joint function.

CLINICAL APPLICATIONS OF HYALURONATE IN HUMANS AND ANIMALS

HA was first proposed as a treatment for patients with arthritic diseases in 1942,[20] but because of its limited availability, research regarding the efficacy of HA as a clinical rheumatologic treatment was not forthcoming. In 1970, reports on the use of HA for the treatment of human osteoarthritis and other arthritic conditions, as well as traumatic and degenerative arthritis in race horses, began to appear.[9,35,37-49] The purpose of this section is to critically review the clinical reports that describe the efficacy of HA for the treatment of human and animal joint diseases.

Types of Clinically Used Forms of HA

To date, three types of sodium HA have been used for ophthalmic surgery: (1) a low-molecular-weight and low-viscosity preparation made from bovine vitreous fluid;[50-53] (2) a more purified, very viscous, and high-molecular-weight preparation made from human umbilical cord or rooster combs;[54,55] and (3) a low-molecular-weight bacterial HA that is used in combination with chondroitin 6-sulfate to form a viscoelastic product.

The second preparation described, made from umbilical cords or, most commonly, rooster combs, has been reported to cause fewer adverse reactions in the eye and has proved to be a valuable ophthalmic surgical adjunct.[56-59] The specific features of this HA preparation are as follows: (1) it is highly purified (i.e., it has a protein content less than 0.5%, and it is sterile and pyrogen free); (2) it is highly concentrated (10–20 mg/ml); and (3) it is viscous (> 20,000 centipoise) and has a high molecular weight ($1-2 \times 10^6$).[35]

Clinical Changes After HA Application

As HA has been shown to influence the inflammatory and repair processes in synovial tissue, it has been speculated that HA plays a positive role in the healing and regeneration of articular cartilage.[35] The clinical research that supports these assumptions involves the treatment of arthritis in horses and the treatment of both traumatic induced degenerative joint disease (of the knees) and idiopathic osteoarthritis in humans.[20,35,37,40,60] The beneficial effect of HA injections in equine joints (observed for periods of time greater than 6 months, which is longer than the expected residence time for HA in the joint) has been a consistent finding in clinical studies. Finally, controlled animal experiments have been performed using experimentally induced cartilage wounds in dog and owl-monkey joints. The results have uniformly supported the notion that joint tissues heal better after HA has been injected into them.[9,61]

Open Clinical Trials in Humans

There have been several open (uncontrolled and unblinded) clinical investigations reported in the literature. In 1974, Peyron and Balazs reported the results of the single injection of HA into the synovial knee joints of 7 patients diagnosed with osteoarthritis.[35] Clinical improvement was excellent for 5 of the 7 patients. The duration of effect in single-injection cases varied from a few days to several months,[35] and the more advanced osteoarthritic joints (i.e., those with associated chondromalacia) were not as responsive to treatment.[26] A 71% favorable response rate was reported in another study using multiple HA injections in 45 osteoarthritic knees of 43 patients.[20] Greater efficacy was noted if the osteoarthrosis was considered to be mild in severity. The presence of joint effusion or gross structural changes resulted in no improvement. These studies obviously suggest that HA has a definite therapeutic effect when applied intraarticularly.

Controlled Clinical Human Experiments

In 1974, Peyron and Balazs also conducted a controlled study without blinding on 8 patients; in this study, a 1-ml injection of each patient's own synovial exudate was administered into his or her osteoarthritic knees. Seven days later the patients were reinjected with 2 ml of HA. Clinical symptoms improved slightly after the control injection but showed marked improvement after the HA injection.[35] In another report, there was significantly greater improvement reported by the 16 patients given knee-joint injections of HA than by the 16 control patients given sham injections (i.e., without blinding).[62]

Similar results on a larger group of patients with knee osteoarthritis (40 joints in 34 patients) have been reported in a double-blind and controlled research study.[60] The data showed that pain relief was more rapid and longer-lasting in the HA group. Although few in number, these controlled experiments offer additional weight to the evidence that HA is an efficacious therapy for some arthritic joints.

Treatment Outcome Considerations

Two issues must be considered when analyzing the results of an HA injection for an arthritic condition. First, how soon after an HA injection will the effect be perceived? Second, how long after the injection will the effect last?

The onset of the effect of HA has been found to be quite variable, ranging from immediate improvement to the need for repeated HA injections. The duration of an effect has also been quite variable. One study reported that the effective duration of a single injection in 7 patients diagnosed with osteoarthritis varied from a few days to several months.[35] In another open clinical

trial, 45 patients with arthritis received 62 injections of HA (into 22 hips and 40 knees). The HA injection effect lasted from 1 week to 12 months, averaging 6 weeks for hips and 10 weeks for knees.[39] A double-blind, placebo-controlled clinical trial found that 40 osteoarthritic–knee-joint patients who received 20 HA and 20 placebo injections had marked symptom relief for 1 month after treatment was discontinued.[60] The most typical duration of the beneficial effect of an HA administration was a few days. Following this period, the patients still reported beneficial effects, but these effects gradually decreased in intensity. This duration effect is logical because HA disappears from the joint cavity within a few days after intraarticular injection.[20,36] Reports of longer-lasting effects cannot be explained by the direct action of HA alone. It is possible that HA functions to increase synovial fluid production, thus improving the joint environment and reestablishing the barrier protecting the synovial membrane and cartilage surfaces.[20] If so, then those patients who have advanced osteoarthritis probably have far too much synovium and too many joint-surface changes for HA to be effective.

HA Versus Corticosteroid Injections

Currently, the most widely accepted injected substance for treating joint pain is corticosteroid. A study was conducted comparing the effectiveness of corticosteroid with that of HA on the temporomandibular joint (TMJ) of human patients with osteoarthritis.[63] This blind, partial cross-over–design study involved a sample of 33 patients who had long-standing TMJ pain as well as tenderness to palpation. The short- and long-term (i.e., 2-year) outcome effects of these injections were analyzed, and both drugs were found to reduce symptoms and signs significantly. No statistically significant difference in effect was found. As a result, investigators concluded that HA might be the best alternative owing to its reduced risk for causing side effects.[64,65]

In an experimental animal model of arthritis, HA injections were found to reduce both the development of deviation in the form of the joint components and the growth of granulation tissues.[66] It was subsequently suggested that early treatment with intraarticular injections of sodium hyaluronate has an inhibitory effect on the joint tissues. This effect is attributed to the high molecular weight of the HA preparation and the consequent mechanical prevention of the development of a fibrinous covering over the articular surfaces and the ingrowth of granulation tissue into the joint space. This effect is probably similar to the results observed in experimental animal wounds treated with HA.[9] In studies of such wounds, no significant difference in the overall severity of the lesions was observed after the corticosteroid or HA injections. There was no statistically significant difference between the two drugs with respect to the presence of radiographic signs even though osteophytes occurred more frequently in joints treated early with corticosteroid.[66]

An uncontrolled and unblinded clinical trial described the outcome results for three patients who received a total of 14 intraarticular injections of a mixture of corticosteroids and HA.[20] Favorable results were reported for this mixture compared with the results of prior treatments using corticosteroid preparations alone. Although no systematic research has been conducted, these findings suggest that injections consisting of a mixture of HA and corticosteroids may produce more positive results than those obtained with the injection of either agent alone.

Side Effects of HA in Human Joints

All drugs must be evaluated for their side effects as well as their therapeutic potential. The fact that HA, a natural component of the connective tissue matrix, has not produced any appreciable deleterious effects on joint tissues would be expected.[67] No clinical signs of inflammation have been observed even though HA injections have been shown to result in transient polymorphonuclear leukocytes, plasma cells, and mononuclear macrophage–like cell infiltration into the synovial membrane.[9,68] The data from various clinical trials indicate that patient tolerance for HA is excellent. This tolerance did not decrease, even after 2–3 injections given at weekly intervals into the same joint. The absence of a reaction indicates that sensitization did not occur.[35] In fact, two separate studies performed multiple (up to 16) repeated HA injections into the hips and the knees without any reported intolerance or side effects.[20,60]

Mild side effects such as stiffness, mild local pain, slight swelling, and heat of the skin at the injection site reported to last from 3 to 36 hours after the injection have been reported.[35,69] However, these side effects are probably due primarily to injection trauma. HA injections have not shown any toxic effect on urine secretion or on blood cell formation.[20,35]

Future Modifications of HA

HA injections for the treatment of human idiopathic and traumatic arthritis are available in some countries. HA has not been overwhelmingly accepted, however, because it is viewed as only a transient palliative treatment without long-lasting effects. Researchers have produced more highly cross-linked HA than oc-

curs naturally. The speculation is that the resulting molecular structure has significantly altered rheologic properties.[26] It has yet to be proved whether the newly engineered, cross-linked HA will result in improved therapeutic activity and longer-lasting effectiveness.

In summary, even though a substantial body of information exists, there are only a few well-designed and well-controlled random clinical trials involving HA use in humans. Clearly, the potential of HA needs further investigation, and more controlled, randomized clinical trials are required in order to honestly evaluate its therapeutic efficacy in different populations with well-defined disease states.

REFERENCES

1. Meyer, K; Palmer, JW. The polysaccharide of the vitreous humor. J Biol Chem (1934), 107:629–634.
2. Swann, DA. Macromolecules in synovial fluid. In: Sokoloff, L, ed. The Joint and Synovial Fluid. New York: Academic Press (1978), 407–439.
3. Fraser, JR; Laurent, TC. Turnover and metabolism of hyaluronan. Ciba Found Symp (1989), 143:41–59.
4. Radin, EL; Paul, IL; Swann, DA; Schottstadt, ES. Lubrication of synovial membrane. Ann Rheum Dis (1971), 30:322–325.
5. Swann, DA; Radin, EL; Nazimiec, M; et al. Role of hyaluronic acid in joint lubrication. Ann Rheum Dis (1974), 33:318–326.
6. Abatangelo, G; Botti, P; Del Bue, M; et al. Intraarticular sodium hyaluronate injections in the Pond-Nuki experimental model of osteoarthritis in dogs: I. Biochemical Results. Clin Orthop (1989), 241:278–285.
7. Miller, D; Stegmann, R, eds. Healon (sodium hyaluronate): A fluid to its use in ophthalmic surgery. New York: John Wiley & Sons (1983).
8. Balazs, EA; Gibbs, DA. The rheological properties and biological function of hyaluronic acid. In: Balazs, EA, ed. Chemistry and Molecular Biology of the Intercellular Matrix. Vol III. New York: Academic Press (1970), 1241.
9. Rydell, N; Balazs, EA. Effect of intra-articular injection of hyaluronic acid on the clinical symptoms of osteoarthritis and on granulation tissue formation. Clin Orthop (1971), 80:25–32.
10. Dahl, LB; Dahl, IMS; Engström-Laurent, A; Granath, K. Concentration and molecular weight of sodium hyaluronate in synovial fluid from patients with rheumatoid arthritis and other arthropathies. Ann Rheum Dis (1985), 44:817.
11. Laurent, TC. Biochemistry of hyaluronan. Acta Otolaryngol Suppl (Stockh) (1987), 442:7–24.
12. Comper, WD; Laurent, TC. Physiological function of connective tissue polysaccharides. Physiol Rev (1978), 58:255–315.
13. Ogston, AG; Phelps, CF. The partition of solutes between buffer solutions and solutions containing hyaluronic acid. Biochem J (1960), 78:827–833.
14. Laurent, TC; Pietruszkiewicz, A. The effect of hyaluronic acid on the sedimentation rate of other substances. Biochim Biophys Acta (1961), 49:258–264.
15. Laurent, TC; Ogston, AG. The interaction between polysaccharides and other macromolecules: The osmotic pressure of mixtures of serum albumin and hyaluronic acid. Biochem J (1963), 89:249–253.
16. Ogston, AG; Stanier, JE. The dimensions of the particle of hyaluronic acid complex in synovial fluid. Biochem J (1951), 49:585–590.
17. Balazs, EA; Bloom, GD; Swann, DA. Fine structure and glycosaminoglycan content of the surface layer of articular cartilage. Fed Proc (1966), 25:1813.
18. Balazs, EA; Darzynkiewicz, Z. The effect of hyaluronic acid on fibroblasts, mononuclear phagocytes and lymphocytes. In: Kulonen, E; Pikkarainen, J, eds. Biology of the Fibroblast, I. New York: Academic Press (1973), 237–252.

19. Toyoshima, H. Influence of synovectomy on articular cartilage of rabbit knee and preventive effects of hyaluronic acid on degenerative changes of the cartilage. J Tokyo Wom Med Coll (1978), 48:20–40.

20. Namiki, O; Toyoshima, H; Morisaki, N. Therapeutic effect of intra-articular injection of high molecular weight hyaluronic acid on osteoarthritis of the knee. Int J Clin Pharmacol Ther Toxicol (1982), 20:501–507.

21. Gibbs, DA; Merrill, EW; Smith, KA; Balazs, EA. Rheology of hyaluronic acid. Biopolymers (1968); 6:777–791.

22. Balazs, EA. Some aspects of the aging and radiation sensitivity of the intercellular matrix with special regard to hyaluronic acid in synovial fluid and vitreous. In: Engel, A, Larsson, T, eds. Thule International Symposium: Aging of Connective and Skeletal Tissue. Stockholm: Nordiska Bokhandelns Forlag (1969), 107–122.

23. Walker, PS; Sikorski, J; Doeson, D; et al. Behavior of synovial fluid on surface of articular cartilage: A scanning electron microscope study. Ann Rheum Dis (1969), 28:1–14.

24. Sommarin, V; Heinegard, D. Specific interaction between cartilage proteoglycan and hyaluronic acid in the chondrocyte cell surface. Biochem J (1983), 214:777.

25. Anatassiades, T; Roberson, W. Modulation of mitogen-dependent lymphocyte stimulation by hyaluronic acid. J Rheumatol (1984), 11:729–734.

26. Balazs, EA; Denlinger, J. Clinical uses of hyaluronan. Ciba Found Symp (1989), 143:265–280.

27. Castor, CW; Prince, RK; Hazelton, MJ. Hyaluronic acid in human synovial effusions: A sensitive indicator of altered connective tissue cell function during inflammation. Arthritis Rheum (1966), 9:783–794.

28. Balazs, EA; Watson, D; Duff, IV; Roseman, S. Hyaluronic acid in synovial fluid: I. Molecular parameters of hyaluronic acid in normal arthritic human fluids. Arthritis Rheum (1968), 10:357–376.

29. McDevitt, CA; Muir, H. Biochemical changes in the cartilage of the knee in experimental and natural osteoarthritis in the dog. J Bone Joint Surg [Am] (1976), 58:94–101.

30. Brandt, KD; Palmoski, MJ; Perricone, E. Aggregation of cartilage proteoglycans. Arthritis Rheum (1976), 19:1308–1314.

31. Thonar, EJ; Sweet, MB; Immelman, AR; Lyons, GF. Hyaluronate in articular cartilage: Age-related changes. Calcif Tissue Res (1978), 26:19–21.

32. Muir, H. Cartilage structure and metabolism and basic changes in degenerative joint disease. Aust N Z J Med (1978), 1:1–5.

33. Vuorio, E; Einola, S; Hakkarainen, S; Penttinen, R. Synthesis of underpolymerized hyaluronic acid by fibroblasts cultured from rheumatoid and non-rheumatoid synovitis. Rheumatol Int (1982), 2:97–102.

34. Ferguson, J; Boyle, JA; Nuki, G. Rheological evidence for the existence of dissociated macromolecular complexes in rheumatoid synovial fluid. Clin Sci (1969), 37:739–750.

35. Peyron, JG; Balazs, EA. Preliminary clinical assessment of Na-hyaluronate injection into human arthritic joints. Pathol Biol (Paris) (1974), 22:731–736.

36. Namiki, O; Toyoshima, H; Morisaki, N; et al. Intraarticular injection of high molecular hyaluronic acid. Orthop Surg (1978), 29:562–568.

37. Butler, J; Rydell, N; Balazs, EA. Hyaluronic acid in synovial fluid: VI. Effect of intra-articular injection of hyaluronic acid on the clinical symptoms of arthritis in track horses. Acta Vet Scand (1970), 11:139–155.

38. Butler, J; Rydell, NW; Balazs, EA. Hyaluronic acid in synovial fluid: VI. Effect of intra-articular injection of hyaluronic acid on the clinical symptoms of arthritis in track horses. Acta Vet Scand (1970), 11:139.

39. Helfet, AJ. Management of osteoarthritis of the knee joint. In: Helfet, AJ, ed. Disorders of the Knee. Philadelphia: JB Lippincott Co. (1974), 175–194.

40. Asheim, A; Lindblad, G. Intra-articular treatment of arthritis in race horses with sodium hyaluronate. Acta Vet Scand (1976), 17:379–394.

41. Gingerich, DA; Auer, JA; Fackelman, GE. Effect of exogenous hyaluronic acid on joint function in experimentally-induced equine osteoarthritis: Dosage titration studies. Res Vet Sci (1981), 30:192–197.

42. McIlwraith, CW. Current concepts in equine degenerative joint disease. J Am Vet Med Assoc (1982), 180:239.

43. Palmoski, MJ; Brandt, KD. Immobilization of the knee prevents osteoarthritis after anterior cruciate ligament transection. Arthritis Rheum (1982), 25:1201.

44. Pezzoli, G; Botti, P; Peri, P. Topical use of hyaluronic acid in the treatment of equine arthropathy. Lecture presented at the Sixth Atti VI National Convention of the Italian Society of Hypology, Salsomaggiore Terme, Italy, June 1983.

45. Pezzoli, G. Role of hyaluronic acid in equine arthropathies. Lecture presented at the International Congress on Hyaluronic Acid in the Treatment of Equine Arthritis/Arthrosis, Parma, Italy, May 1984.

46. Sakamoto, T; Mizuno, S; Miyazaki, K; et al. Biological fate of sodium hyaluronate (SPH): (1) Studies on distribution, metabolism and excretion of ^{14}C-SPH in rabbits after intra-articular administration. Pharmacometrics (1984), 28:375.

47. Bragantini, A; Cassini, M; De Bastiani, G; et al. Controlled single-blind trial of intra-articularly injected hyaluronic acid (Hyalgan) in osteoarthritis of the knee. Clin Tri J (1987), 24:333–340.

48. Punzi, L; Schiavon, F; Ramonda, R; et al. Intraarticular hyaluronic acid in the treatment of inflammatory and noninflammatory knee effusions. Curr Ther Res (1988), 43:643–647.

49. Punzi, L; Schiavon, F; Cavasin, F; et al. The influence of intra-articular hyaluronic acid on PGE2 and cAMP of synovial fluid. Clin Exp Rheumatol (1989), 7:247–250.

50. Hruby, K. Hyaluronsäure als Glaskörperersatz bei Netzhautablösung. Klin Mbl Augenheilk (1961), 138:484–496.

51. Hruby K. Substitution du corps vitre. Glaskörperersatz. Substitutes of vitreous body. In: Modern Problems of Ophthalmology, VIII. Basel and New York: S. Karger (1969), 128–135.

52. Moreau, PG; Rouher, F; Plane, C. L'acide hyaluronique dans la chirurgie du vitré. Ann Oculist (1968), 201:193–202.

53. Girod, P; Rouchy, JP. L'acide hyaluronique dans la chirurgie du corps vitré: Réflexions à propos de 24 cas. Ann Oculist (1970), 203:25–40.

54. Swann, DA. Studies on hyaluronic acid: I. The preparation and properties of rooster comb hyaluronic acid. Biochim Biophys Acta (1968a), 156:17–30.

55. Swann, DA. Studies on hyaluronic acid. II. The protein component(s) of rooster comb hyaluronic acid. Biochim Biophys Acta (1968b), 160:96–105.

56. Regnault, F. Acide hyaluronique intracitreen et cryocoagulation dans le traitement des formes graves de décollement de la rétine. Bull Soc Francaise Ophtalmol (1971), 84:106–112.

57. Balazs, EA; Freeman, MI; Klöti R; et al. Hyaluronic acid and the replacement of the vitreous and aqueous humor. In: Streiff, EB. Modern Problems of Ophthalmology. Basel, Switzerland: S. Karger (1972), 3–21.

58. Algvere, P. Intravitreal injection of high-molecular-weight hyaluronic acid in retinal detachment. Acta Ophthalmol (Copenh) (1971), 49:975–976.

59. Klöti R. Hyaluronsäure als Glaskörpersubstituent. Ophthalmologica (1972), 165:351–359.

60. Grecomoro, G; Martorana, U; Di Marco, C. Intra-articular treatment with sodium hyaluronate in gonarthrosis: A controlled clinical trial versus placebo. Pharmatherapeutica (1987), 5:137–141.

61. Schiavinato, A; Lini, E; Guidolin, D; et al. Intraarticular sodium hyaluronate injections in the Pond-Nuki experimental model of osteoarthritis in dogs: II. Morphological findings. Clin Orthop (1989), 241:286–299.

62. Weiss, C; Balazs, EA; St. Onge, R; Denlinger, JL. Clinical studies of the intraarticular injection of Healon (sodium hyaluronate) in the treatment of osteoarthritis of human knees. Semin Arthritis Rheum (1981), 11:143–144.

63. Kopp, S; Wenneberg, B; Haraldson, T; et al. The short-term effect of intra-articular injections of sodium hyaluronate and corticosteroid on temporomandibular joint pain and dysfunction. J Oral Maxillofac Surg (1985), 43:429–435.

64. Chandler, GN; Wright, V. Deleterious effect of intra-articular hydrocortisone. Lancet (1958), 2:661.

65. Sevastik, J. Lemperg, R. Lokala bendestruktioner efter intraartikulär injektion av kortikosteroider. Nord Med (1969), 82:949.

66. Mejersjö, C; Kopp, S. Effect of corticosteroid and sodium hyaluronate on induced joint lesions in the guinea-pig knee. Int J Oral Maxillofac Surg (1987), 16:194–201.

67. Falk, J. Repeated injections of sodium hyaluronate into the knee joints of dogs. Internal Report, Pharmacia AB, Sweden Report (1974), L 287 C 8.

68. Wigren, A; Wik, O; Falk, J. Repeated intra-articular implantation of hyaluronic acid: An experimental study in normal and immobilized adult rabbit knee joints. Ups J Med Sci Suppl (1975).

69. Kopp, S; Wenneberg, B. Injektion av healonid i käkled: En preliminär rapport. Department of Stomatognathic Physiology, Göteborg University. Report Series No. 22, August 1979.

Nineteen

The Histologic Basis and Clinical Implications for Temporomandibular Joint Adaptation

CAROL A. BIBB, Ph.D., D.D.S.
ANDREW G. PULLINGER, D.D.S., M.Sc.

The concept of the adaptive temporomandibular joint (TMJ) has been a useful model for understanding the relationships between structure and function in the TMJ. This perspective has encouraged the development of a biologic rationale for diagnosis and treatment decisions and has led to a better interpretation of clinical imaging. To refine this concept, the following questions must be answered: What tissues and cells are responsible for the hypothesized adaptive responses? Can histologic stages of adaptation be identified? Is it possible to identify histologic markers of irreversible stages that would imply progression and breakdown? The research reviewed in this chapter addresses the first question and supports speculation about the remaining two. These issues are pertinent to an understanding of the sequelae of TMJ arthroscopic procedures.

IMPORTANT HISTOLOGIC FEATURES

The microanatomy of the TMJ articular tissues has been described in animal models[1-3] as well as human autopsy material from both young adult[4-6] and elderly populations.[4,7,8] The mammalian jaw joint has special-

ized features that distinguish it from most other synovial joints. These unusual features include articular surfaces of fibrous connective tissue (rather than hyaline cartilage) and an articular disk that completely divides the joint into separate compartments.

The tissue layers covering the condyle and temporal component of the TMJ are qualitatively similar.[4,7] Beginning at the articular surface, these layers are (1) the articular zone of fibrous connective tissue, (2) the proliferation zone of undifferentiated mesenchymal (UM) cells, and (3) the cartilage zone (Fig. 19–1). Together these noncalcified tissues are often referred to as the *articular soft tissue* in order to emphasize the difference between them and the underlying bone. Previous studies have described the variation in overall soft tissue thickness and have attributed it to loading differences across the articular surfaces.[7,9] The absence of an identifiable UM cell layer has also been described as a marker for adverse loading.[10-12]

In contrast to the soft tissues covering the condyle and temporal component, in young adult humans the articular disk is composed of fibrous connective tissue; variable conversion to fibrocartilage occurs with increased age.[7] The disk, which lacks a proliferation zone of UM cells, has been considered the passive joint

163

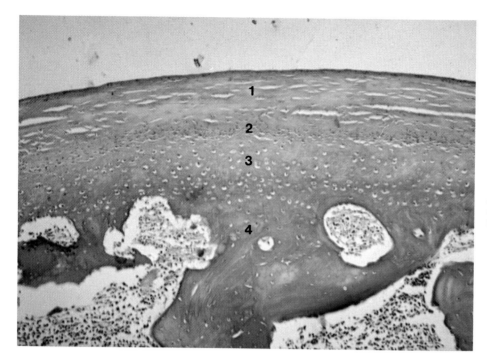

FIGURE 19–1. Photomicrograph of the superior sector of a condyle from a 30-year-old male. The tissue layers are (1) the articular zone of fibrous connective tissue, (2) the proliferation zone of undifferentiated mesenchymal (UM) cells, (3) the cartilage zone, and (4) compact bone.

component and to have a greater ability to accommodate than to adapt.[12,13]

Our studies[14–16] have taken a more detailed look at human TMJ histology in young adults. The population group ranging in age from 16 to 38 years is considered clinically relevant for study.[17] We found that it is conceptually useful to divide the joint into three regions: 1) the proliferative cartilage zone of the condyle and temporal component; 2) the articular–synovial-lining tissue system; and 3) the articular disk and posterior attachment.

The Proliferative Cartilage Zone

The UM cells of the proliferation zone have been identified as the precursor cells of the cartilage zone on the basis of autoradiographic studies in animal models.[2,3] The same studies reported that the articular zone of fibrous connective tissue was renewed independently of UM cell activity and at a much slower rate. Hansson and coworkers[9–11] used observations on human autopsy material to suggest that the UM cells lay down additional cartilage in response to functional loading, thereby producing changes in soft tissue thickness and in articular surface shape termed *deviation in form* (DIF). It was further hypothesized that this process may lead to the depletion of the UM cell population, a phenomenon that Hansson[12] considered a predegenerative condition. Historically, support for the UM cell hypothesis comes from reports of a statistically significant inverse relationship between overall soft tissue thickness and UM cell presence.[10,11,18] How-

ever, these studies did not present the strength of this association. We have reexamined this issue and hypothesize that the contribution of UM cells to articular tissue maintenance may have been overstated.

In our histologic model of young adult TMJs, UM cell presence was not related to soft tissue thickness, cartilage thickness, or DIF in the condyle, posterior slope, or fossa of the temporal component.[6,19] The only exception was a moderate inverse correlation between soft tissue thickness and UM cell presence observed in the articular eminence location of the temporal component. In the young adult joints, complete absence of UM cells was common but there was no associated evidence of degeneration. If UM cell depletion is viewed as a predegenerative condition, the high frequency of UM cell depletion in our results would predict a much higher prevalence of arthrosis than has been shown in epidemiologic population studies. In addition, DIF described from direct observation of articular surface irregularity did not correlate with increased soft tissue thickness.[16] Since earlier definitions of DIF were based on increased soft tissue thickness, the current authors believe there is a need for an improved DIF definition.

Nevertheless, one should not discount the importance of activity in the proliferative cartilage zone in moderating osseous irregularities. Even dramatic osseous concavities (Fig. 19–2) in the condyles of young adults were usually compensated by an increase in the overlying cartilage.[15] The long-term outcome of this type of response cannot be determined from cross-sectional studies but is presumably dependent on activity at the cartilage-bone boundary. Certainly, when viewing TMJ radiographs, overinterpreting bone changes as osteoarthrosis may result in the ignoring of a successful adaptation response by the soft tissue.

We propose that other processes in addition to UM cell activity must be involved in TMJ articular tissue dynamics. For example, the UM cell hypothesis does not take into account events at the cartilage-bone boundary representing the histologic interface between the soft tissue and the bone. Early activity at this interface may modify the cartilage layer by bone deposition, thus moderating an increase in soft tissue thickness. Further study of the tissue dynamics at this interface may prove useful for the staging of arthrosis, particularly in the early stages of the disease and prior to obvious bone loss.

The Articular–Synovial-Lining Tissue System

The articular zone of fibrous connective tissue represents the actual articular surface of the condyle and temporal component; it is also the tissue directly visualized by arthroscopy. Previous authors have considered this layer to be the passive component of the soft tissue that varies little in thickness.[2,8,10]

In our studies of young adult joints, the fibrous connective tissue layer contributed to overall soft tissue thickness variations as much as did the cartilage layer and was always present even when a cartilage layer was not evident.[16] The absence of cartilage in the depth of the fossa and in the posterior sector of the condyle—regions presumably not subject to functional loading—was frequently observed. These observations led to the conclusion that cartilage is the histologic marker for loading, whereas the fibrous connective tissue layer is ultimately responsible for maintenance of an intact articular surface. This conclusion is dramatically illustrated by a condyle in which an osseous defect was compensated by only fibrous connective tissue[20] (Figure 19–3).

Around each joint compartment there was a lining of connective tissue that was continuous across the articular surfaces and around the joint recesses. Synovial tissue was present in the recesses, with the areolar type localized to the upper posterior and the lower anterior recesses (Fig. 19–4). The lower posterior and the upper anterior recesses had fibrous synovial tissue (Fig. 19–5). The upper anterior recess characteristically presented as a cleft in the fibrous connective tissue (Fig. 19–5). There was no obvious boundary, but rather a gradual transition in histologic appearance between the articular fibrous connective tissue and the tissue lining the recesses. It is therefore not surprising that during direct arthroscopic visualization boundaries between adjacent tissues are defined as much by location as by appearance.[21]

Another consistent observation in our study was that functionally juxtaposed articular surfaces of the condyle, the disk, and the temporal component were histologically identical in 19 of 20 joints examined.[20] In other words, the opposing articulating surface tissues were indistinguishable at sufficiently high magnification (Fig. 19–6). The single exception was a joint with a displaced disk whose histologic character did not match the opposing articular surfaces of the condyle and the temporal component. Two important questions are raised by these observations: Are the histologically

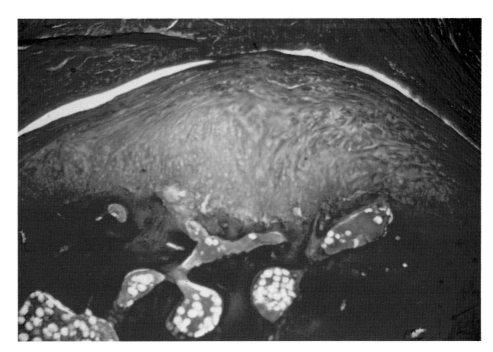

FIGURE 19–2. Photomicrograph of an osseous concavity in the superior aspect of a condyle from a 32-year-old male. Note that the concavity is filled with fibrocartilage and that there is a smooth, intact articular surface. This concavity measured 1.24 mm from the articular surface to the cartilage-bone boundary. (From Baldioceda, F; Bibb, CA; Pullinger, AG. Distribution and histologic character of osseous concavities in mandibular condyles of young adults. J Craniomandib Dis Fac Oral Pain (1990), 4:147–153.)

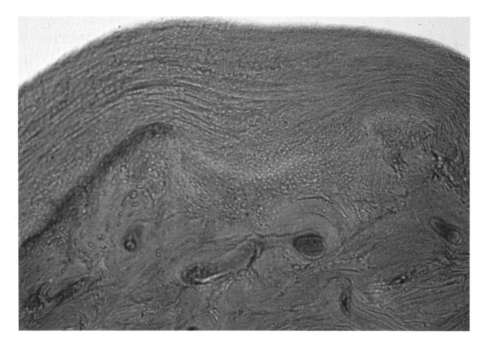

FIGURE 19–3. Photomicrograph of an osseous concavity in the superior aspect of a condyle from a 35-year-old female. This concavity is 1 mm deep and covered with fibrous connective tissue with no identifiable cartilage zone or UM cells. (From Baldioceda, F; Bibb, CA; Pullinger, AG. Distribution and histologic character of osseous concavities in mandibular condyles of young adults. J Craniomandib Dis Fac Oral Pain (1990), 4:147–153.)

similar surfaces necessary for nonadherence of surfaces brought into functional contact? Also, does the exception represent a recent disk displacement that over time will acquire the same fibrous character in response to altered function?

We propose the term articular–synovial–lining tissue system to emphasize the continuity of the compartment-lining tissues.[20] It is hypothesized that the function of this system is to maintain intact and nonadherent articular surfaces between functionally juxtaposed joint components. Within the system, the proportion that is synovial or articular may depend on location and loading. An intriguing possibility is that all of the lining tissues be considered synovial tissue based on a functional definition of nonadherence.[22]

The Articular Disk and the Posterior Attachment

The potential for histologic adaptation of the articular disk posterior attachment is very pertinent to the success of arthroscopically treated closed-lock. The articular disks in 80–92% of the closed-lock patients

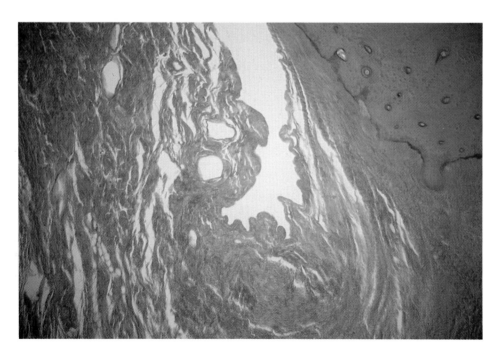

FIGURE 19–4. Photomicrograph of the upper posterior recess with areolar synovial tissue. Note the loose connective tissue with a large surface area and vascular bed.

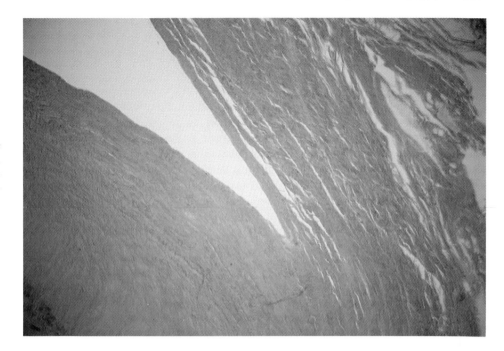

FIGURE 19–5. Photomicrograph of the upper anterior recess with fibrous synovial tissue. This recess has the histologic appearance of a cleft rather than a distinct pouch as is seen in Figure 20–4.

have been reported to remain in an anterior relationship to the condyle following arthroscopy, yet in most cases there was a significant improvement in disk movement and jaw function.[23,24] Consequently, in this position the condyle rests on the posterior attachment area. The question confronting the clinician is whether the posterior attachment will become compressed and perforated, leading to degenerative joint disease, or will successfully adapt by virtue of a fibrous response. In cases of disk displacement, pseudodisk formation by fibrous metaplasia of the retrodiscal tissues is fre-

quently hypothesized based on reports of fibrous tissue in the retrodiscal area.[25]

In a study of 50 young adult TMJs, the relationship between the histology of the posterior attachment to disk position and disk morphology was examined.[26] In 24% of the specimens the disks were displaced; this permitted comparison of tissue characterization to the normally positioned disks. Fifty-eight percent of the disks were biconcave, and the remainder were classified as (1) biconcave and elongated, (2) biconcave, elongated, and flattened, or (3) biconcave and deformed.

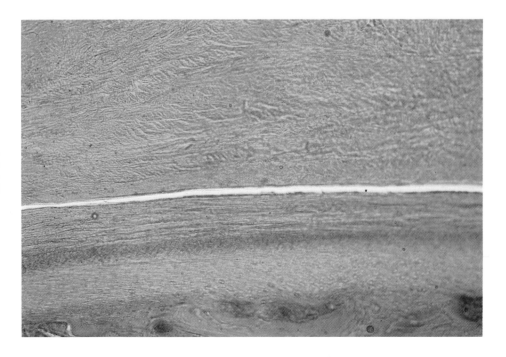

FIGURE 19–6. At high magnification the functionally juxtaposed articular surfaces of the condyle (below) and disk (above) are identical in histologic character.

All deformed disks were displaced, but not all displaced disks were deformed.

Bilamination of the posterior attachment has been traditionally described as the combination of an inferior ligament and a superior lamina of looser and elastic tissue. This original description of the so-called bilaminar zone was based on a sample size of only two histologic specimens.[27] In a study of 20 joints the bilaminar zone was not a consistent anatomic feature, as only one third of the specimens showed definitive bilamination.[26] We believe that the concept of a bilaminar zone is misleading and that it is more appropriate to consider the *degree* of bilamination.

In our studies[26] the displaced disks were characterized by a lack of bilamination and generalized posterior attachment fibrosis. However, this did not distinguish them from normally positioned disks, two thirds of which also showed posterior attachment fibrosis. This illustrates the fact that fibrosis of the posterior attachment is not exclusively the sequela of disk displacement, but rather is a common anatomic feature independent of disk position. The proportion of fibrous to elastic tissue in the posterior attachment may be more a reflection of the functional jaw movement characteristics of each individual.[28]

Figure 19–7 shows an apparently successfully adapted displaced disk with favorable posterior attachment fibrosis, elongation of the fibrous part of the disk, and disk flattening. The factors contributing to a successful adaptive response in the posterior attachment remain obscure. The traditional approach of clinicians has been to unload the retrodiscal tissues in joints with posterior attachment impingement. However, an alternate approach in which fibrous change is

stimulated through functional loading may be more correct.[29] Another interesting possibility is that joints with posterior attachment fibrosis prior to disk displacement may be most likely to accommodate a change in the relationship between the disk and the condyle. This kind of information may be obtainable during pretreatment imaging using magnetic resonance, although there will be some inherent difficulty in differentiating the limit of the fibrous part of the disk from the posterior attachment.

SUMMARY

Three sites in the young adult TMJ with potential for histologic adaptation have been described. The condyle and temporal component have a proliferative cartilage zone with the capacity to moderate osseous irregularities. Overinterpretation of all radiographic bone changes as osteoarthrosis may overlook a successful adaptation response by the soft tissue. Conversely, it is anticipated that the cartilage-bone interface is the location of histologic markers useful in staging the early phases of arthrosis. The proposed articular–synovial-lining tissue system is responsible for maintaining intact, nonadherent articular surfaces independent of changes in the underlying cartilage, the underlying bone, and the disk position. An understanding of the surface characteristics responsible for nonadherence is expected to provide insight into the mechanisms of adhesion that cause or maintain joint locking. The posterior attachment of the articular disk has much greater potential to adapt histologically to changes in disk position than has been previously thought. We

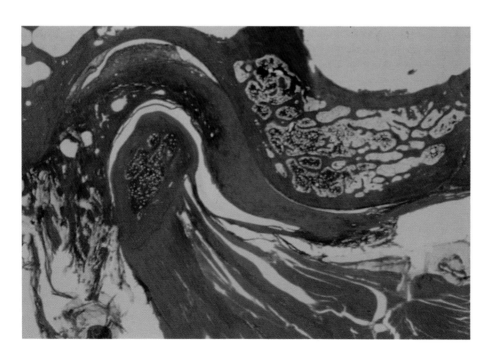

FIGURE 19–7. Photograph of a histologic section from a joint of a 35-year-old female. Note the disk elongation and flattening and posterior attachment fibrosis. (Courtesy of Dr. W. K. Solberg.)

believe that the morphologic and histologic information potentially available from magnetic resonance imaging has been underutilized and has overemphasized disk position. The available histologic information suggests that degenerative joint disease is not an inevitable consequence of disk displacement and that late bone changes may frequently be an adaptive response and not articular breakdown.

REFERENCES

1. Oberg, T. Morphology, growth, and matrix formation in the mandibular joint of the guinea pig. Thesis, Trans R School Dent, Stockholm, 1964.
2. Blackwood, HJJ. Growth of the mandibular condyle of the rat studied with tritiated thymidine. Arch Oral Biol (1966), 11:493–500.
3. Oberg, T; Fajers, CM; Lohmander, S; Friberg, V. Autoradiographic studies with H-3 thymidine on cell proliferation and differentiation in the mandibular joint of young guinea pigs. Odontol Rev (1967), 18:327–344.
4. Carlsson, GE; Oberg, T. Remodeling of the temporomandibular joints. Oral Sci Rev (1974), 6:53–86.
5. Wright, DM; Moffett, BC. The postnatal development of the human temporomandibular joint. Am J Anat (1974), 141:235–250.
6. Baldioceda, F. Prediction of articular soft tissue configuration in human mandibular condyles. Master of Science Thesis, University of California, Los Angeles, 1988.
7. Moffett, BC; Johnson, LC; McCabe, JB; Askew, HC. Articular remodeling in the adult human temporomandibular joint. Am J Anat (1964), 115:119–142.
8. Blackwood, HJJ. Cellular remodeling in articular tissue. J Dent Res (1966), 45:480–489.
9. Hansson, T; Oberg, T; Carlsson; GE; Kopp, S. Thickness of the soft tissue layers and the articular disc in the temporomandibular joint. Acta Odontol Scand (1977), 35:77–83.
10. Hansson, TL; Nordstrom, B. Thickness of the soft tissue layers and articular disc in temporomandibular joints with deviation in form. Acta Odontol Scand (1977), 35:281–288.
11. Lubsen, CC; Hansson; TL; Nordstrom; BB; Solberg, WK. Histomorphometric analysis of cartilage and subchondral bone in mandibular condyles of young human adults at autopsy. Arch Oral Biol (1985), 30:129–136.
12. Hansson, TL. Current concepts about the temporomandibular joint. J Prosthet Dent (1986), 55:370–371.
13. Hansson, TL; Oberg; T. Arthrosis and deviation in form in the temporomandibular joint. Acta Odontol Scand (1977), 35:161–174.
14. Baldioceda, F; Pullinger, AG; Bibb, CA. Relationship of condylar bone profiles and dental factors to articular soft tissue thickness. J Craniomandib Dis Fac Oral Pain (1990), 4:71–79.
15. Baldioceda, F; Bibb, CA; Pullinger, AG. Distribution and histologic character of osseous concavities in mandibular condyles of young adults. J Craniomandib Dis Fac Oral Pain (1990), 4:147–153.
16. Pullinger, AG; Baldioceda, F; Bibb, CA. Relationship of TMJ articular soft tissue to underlying bone in young adult condyles. J Dent Res (1990), 69:1512–1518.
17. Pullinger, A; Seligman, D. TMJ osteoarthrosis: A differentiation of diagnostic subgroups by symptom history and demographics. J Craniomandib Dis Fac Oral Pain (1988), 1:251–256.
18. Bibb, C; Nordstrom, B; Hansson, TL; Solberg, WK. Soft tissue thickness in temporal components of young adult TMJs. J Dent Res (1984), 63:228.
19. Bibb, C; Pullinger, AG; Baldioceda, F. Undifferentiated mesenchymal cell distribution and tissue relationships in mandibular condyles. J Dent Res (1988), 67:402.
20. Bibb, C; Pullinger, A; Baldioceda, F. The articular–synovial lining tissue system in young adult TMJs. J Dent Res (1989), 68:229.
21. Bibb, CA; Pullinger, AG; Baldioceda, F; et al. TMJ comparative imaging: Diagnostic efficacy of arthroscopy compared to tomography and arthrography. Oral Surg Oral Med Oral Pathol (1989), 68:352–359.
22. Henderson, B; Edwards, JCW. The Synovial Lining in Health and Disease. London: Chapman and Hall (1987), 42.
23. Montgomery, MT; Van Sickels, JE; Harms, SE; Thrash, WJ. Arthroscopic TMJ surgery: Effects on signs, symptoms, and disc position. J Oral Maxillofac Surg (1989), 47:1263–1271.
24. Moses, JJ; Sartoris, D; Glass, R; et al. The effect of arthroscopic surgical lysis and lavage of the superior joint space on TMJ disc position and mobility. J Oral Maxillofac Surg (1989), 47:674–678.
25. Scapino, RP. Histopathology associated with malposition of the human temporomandibular joint disc. Oral Surg Oral Med Oral Pathol (1983), 55:382–397.
26. Baldioceda, F; Bibb, CA; Pullinger, AG. Morphologic variability in the human TMJ disc and posterior attachment. J Dent Res (1989), 68:229.
27. Rees, LA. The structure and function of the mandibular joint. Br Dent J (1954), 96:125–133.
28. Moffet, B. Personal communication, 1985.
29. Hahn, B. Personal communication, 1989.

Twenty
Synovial Fluid Pressure

JEROLD S. GOLDBERG, D.D.S.

The significance of disk position in temporomandibular joint (TMJ) disease has been questioned owing to magnetic resonance imaging (MRI) findings and arthroscopic observations. MRI studies have demonstrated displaced disks in over 25% of normal subjects.[1] Imaging studies have also revealed that disks surgically repositioned into proper anatomic position were displaced after surgery. Postoperative disk position did not necessarily influence patients' symptoms, and arthroscopic manipulations have resulted in the elimination of pain and dysfunction, even though disk position did not change.[2] Arthroscopic examination has also revealed that there may be a significant structural alteration in the TMJ, consisting of adhesions, synovitis, and chondromalacia, without the disk appearing displaced in preoperative imaging studies. It is, therefore, evident from these findings that disk position is not the sole factor involved in internal derangement and that it is important that we better understand the function of the TMJ in health and in disease states.

The role of synovial fluid in joint function is obviously important because it plays a primary role in the nutrition and the lubrication of articular surfaces. Various forms of pressure on articular surfaces are probably mediated by synovial fluid, and increases in the volume of synovial fluid or decreases in joint volume can result in increased intraarticular pressure. Therefore, the synovial fluid pressure in normal and diseased joints has been studied for some time. Studies have been performed on animals or on human subjects with rheumatoid arthritis or other pathologies resulting in joint effusion. Investigations involving the TMJ and synovial fluid pressure have been carried out in a combined effort between the Departments of Oral and Maxillofacial Surgery and Orthodontics at Case Western Reserve University in Cleveland, Ohio. These studies are discussed after a review of other literature on synovial fluid pressure.

It has been demonstrated by Reeves,[3] Guyton and associates,[4] Levick,[5] and others that synovial fluid pressure is slightly subatmospheric. These negative pressures are thought to play a role in normal joint lubrication and nutrition, as they would tend to draw fluid and nutrients into the joint space. Active transport mechanisms are probably necessary to remove fluid and debris from the joint. Joint motion and exercise increase synovial fluid pressure, but in normal joints the pressure quickly returns to baseline when these activities are stopped. The rate at which pressures are reduced would indicate significant compliance within the system.

In disease states characterized by inflammation and joint effusion such as rheumatoid arthritis, synovial fluid pressure is sustained at markedly high levels. The influence of increases in articular pressure observed in inflamed joints has been studied by several authors. Levick and colleagues[6] have shown that the permeability of synovium increases at higher intraarticular pressures. McDonald and Levick[7] and Stevens and coworkers[8] have investigated the structural changes that are associated with the increased permeability that is seen with increased articular pressure. They demonstrated that increased pressures are associated with thinner synovial membranes possessing an increased interstitium exposed to the joint surface. With this change, the capillary depth from the synovial lining surface of the joint was reduced.

Blake and colleagues[9] showed that exercise can cause large increases in intraarticular pressures in inflamed

171

knee joints; these pressures can exceed capillary perfusion pressures and, at times, even systolic blood pressures. In a chronic disease state, such as rheumatoid arthritis, exchange vessels were found to be buried deep below the synovial surface and in such reduced numbers that oxygen transfer was decreased. Such a condition may lead to intraarticular hypoxia. McDonald and Levick[7] showed that small increases in intraarticular pressure result in only mild compression of synovial capillaries; they postulated, however, that at higher intraarticular pressures, such as those observed in knee effusions, this flattening could well progress to collapse or reduce blood flow within the synovial tissues.

It has been speculated that reduced synovial blood flow, which is seen at increases of 10–30 mm Hg, may cause ischemia and tissue damage and subsequently lead to fibrosis of the joint capsule. An increase in joint pressure can be caused not only by an increase in volume but also by a reduction in the compliance of the capsule, resulting in increased pressure within the capsule.

Jayson and Dixon[10] demonstrated that there is a relationship between intraarticular pressure and associated muscle function. During quadriceps function, patients with existing inflammation had a significant increase in intraarticular pressure associated with muscle function. Gebarek and coworkers[11] showed that increased synovial fluid pressure due to effusion inhibited the function of knee extensor muscle.

Patients with inflamed joints have abnormalities consistent with oxidative damage. Blake and associates[9] postulated that the activity that generates reactive oxygen species (ROS) may play a role in joint disease. Although inflamed synovial fluid tension is low, ROS may be generated between episodes of acute ischemia when oxygen tension again rises; Blake and associates have termed this phenomenon *hypoxic-reperfusion* injury. These observations, which concern joint hypoxia at increased pressure, synovial reaction to pressure, the formation of potentially detrimental ROS, and the relationship between muscle and joint pressure, are certainly important in understanding the function and the disease process within synovial joints.

Roth and colleagues[12] investigated synovial fluid pressure in the TMJ of domestic pigs. A wick catheter was inserted into the superior joint space. The wick unit was connected to a pressure transducer, which fed output to an amplifier and recorded results on a chart. It was determined that the resting synovial fluid pressure of the TMJ was similar to that reported in knees in humans and in experimental animals (a mean of approximately −4 mm Hg). An additional experiment was carried out to reinforce the findings of subatmospheric pressure. A 24-gauge needle was filled to the hub with fluid. Placing the needle into subcutaneous

tissue caused no measurable change in the amount of fluid in the needle. However, as soon as the needle was placed within the joint space the fluid immediately disappeared from the needle into the joint space. These findings support the hypothesis that pressure gradients provide pathways for fluid and nutrients to enter the joint and that most likely an active transport mechanism is necessary for the movement of fluid into the joint and debris out of it.

While the animal was anesthetized, the jaw was manually placed in various positions. Moving the jaw into an opening position caused an increase in pressure of approximately 6 mm Hg. Protruding the jaw and producing lateral excursions resulted in similar increases in pressure. However, in one instance, when the mandible was moved into lateral excursion away from the joint being measured (i.e., the balancing side) the synovial fluid pressure was considerably higher—approximately 12 mm Hg (Fig. 20–1). In all cases, when the jaw was moved into a particular position the increase in pressure was transient and diminished to the original resting value within 2–3 minutes. In the conscious animal the resting pressure was still subatmospheric but slightly higher than that in the anesthetized animal. There were similar increases in pressure with various jaw movements. One interesting phenomenon observed in the conscious animal was that there was an initial decrease in synovial fluid pressure before the increase in pressure observed in the anesthetized animals. This initial decrease in pressure upon initiation of jaw movement has been observed in other joints. It may be that the action of muscles attached to or adjacent to the capsule may alter the volume of the capsule on initial contraction and, therefore, decrease pressure.

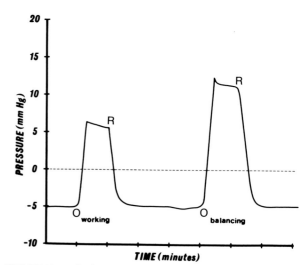

FIGURE 20–1. Fluid pressure response to operator-induced "working" and "balancing" side shifts. (From Roth, TE; Goldberg, JS; Behrents, RG. Synovial fluid pressure determination in the temporomandibular joint. Oral Surg Oral Med Oral Pathol (1984), 57:586.)

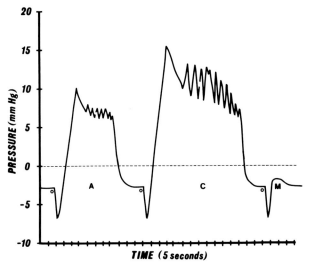

FIGURE 20–2. Fluid pressure response during unassisted mastication. An initial decrease in pressure occurs during unassisted opening. (A: mastication of a soft apple; C: mastication of hard candy; M: A marshmallow that is swallowed without being chewed.) (From Roth, TE; Goldberg, JS; Behrents, RG. Synovial fluid pressure determination in the temporomandibular joint. Oral Surg Oral Med Oral Pathol (1984), 57:587.)

The animals were also fed food of various textures (Fig. 20–2). Synovial fluid pressures increased upon mastication and generally were higher when they were chewing hard food than when chewing soft food. These findings are entirely consistent with experiments with other joints.

Ward and associates[13] later repeated these experi-

ments on an additional set of animals. The initial findings concerning negative resting pressure and the influence of jaw movements on pressure were reproduced. However, Ward and associates noted an initial decrease in pressure on jaw movement in anesthetized animals similar to that which Roth and colleagues observed only in conscious animals.

Two additional experiments were carried out to evaluate the influence of protrusive and retrusive mandibular movements on synovial fluid levels. A ramped splint fastened to the teeth of one animal caused its mandible to move posteriorly (a posterior positioning appliance). A second animal's splint was ramped in such a way so as to cause the mandible to move anteriorly (an anterior positioning appliance). The synovial fluid pressure was measured in both of these animals during and after the time of splint placement.

In the animal with the anterior positioning splint, synovial pressure increased to approximately 10 mm Hg, but diminished to resting pressures over approximately 2 1/2 hours (Fig. 20–3). This finding did not support the theories about functional appliances, which suggest that they work owing to sustained intraarticular pressure.

In the animal that had a splint that moved the mandible posteriorly, the synovial fluid pressure in-

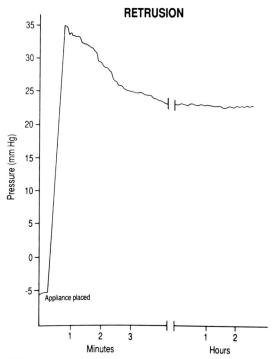

FIGURE 20–4. Synovial fluid pressure response when the posterior positioning splint was placed. Peak pressure was approximately 35 mm Hg, with pressure decaying to approximately 23 mm Hg. Pressure recordings never indicated a return to the original baseline value. (From Ward, DM; Behrents, RG; Goldberg, JS. Temporomandibular synovial fluid pressure response to altered mandibular positions. Am J Dentofac Orthop (1990), 98:26.)

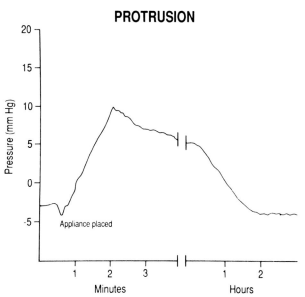

FIGURE 20–3. Synovial fluid pressure response when the anterior positioning splint was placed. Peak pressure is approximately 10 mm Hg, with pressure decaying over the course of 2 hours. (From Ward, DM; Behrents, RG; Goldberg, JS. Temporomandibular synovial fluid pressure response to altered mandibular positions. Am J Dentofac Orthop (1990), 98:25.)

creased to 35 mm Hg immediately after splint placement. The pressure decreased to about 23 mm Hg and stayed at about this level for as long as the splint was in the mouth (Fig. 20–4). This finding supported theories that occlusions that posteriorly position condyles may cause increased pressure and joint disease.

These initial attempts to investigate synovial fluid pressure in the TMJ have yielded useful information. Further investigations to reproduce results and expand knowledge must be performed. If similar findings in the TMJ and knee continue to result, it may be possible to apply information about one joint to the other. As more is known about joint function, hopefully action can be taken to prevent and influence the course of synovial joint diseases.

REFERENCES

1. Kircos, LT; Ortendahl, DA; Mark, AS; Arakawa, M. Magnetic resonance imaging of the TMJ disk in asymptomatic volunteers. J Oral Maxillofac Surg (1987), 45:852–854.
2. Farole, A; Barry, T. Comparison of pre- and postoperative MR imaging of internal derangement of the temporomandibular joint: Correlation with clinical symptoms. RSHA Sci Program (1990), 17:127.
3. Reeves, B. Negative pressures in knee joints. Nature (1966), 212:1046.
4. Guyton, AC; Granger, HJ; Taylor, AE. Interstitial fluid pressure. Physiol Rev (1971), 51:527–563.
5. Levick, JR. The influence of hydrostatic pressure on trans-synovial fluid movement and on capsular expansion of the knee. J Physiol (Lond) (1979), 289:69–82.
6. Levick, JR; Knight, AD. Osmotic flows across the blood–joint barrier. Ann Rheum Dis (1987), 46:534–539.
7. McDonald, JH; Levick, RJ. Pressure-induced deformations of the interstitial route across synovium and its relation to hydraulic conductance. J Rheumatol (1990), 17:341–348.
8. Stevens, CR; Reuell, PA; Blake, DR; Leuck, JR. Synovial vascular morphometry suggests that a state of chronic hypoxia exists in rheumatoid joints (abstract). Bone & Joint Research Unit, London Hospital Medical College and Department of Physiology, St. George's Hospital Medical School.
9. Blake, DR; Unsworth, J; Outhwaite, JM; et al. Hypoxic-perfusion injury in the inflamed human joint. Lancet (1989), 12:289–292.
10. Jayson, MI; Dixon, AS. Intra-articular pressure in rheumatoid arthritis of the knee: 3. Pressure changes during joint use. Ann Rheum Dis (1970), 29:401–408.
11. Gebarek, P; Moritz, V; Wollheim, FA. Joint capsule stiffness in knee arthritis. Relationship to intraarticular volume, hydrostatic pressure, and extensor muscle function. J Rheumatol (1989), 16:1351–1358.
12. Roth, TE; Goldberg, JS; Behrents, RG. Synovial fluid pressure demonstration in the temporomandibular joint. Oral Surg Oral Med Oral Pathol (1984), 57:583–588.
13. Ward, DM; Behrents, RG; Goldberg, JS. Temporomandibular synovial fluid pressure response to altered mandibular positions. Am J Dentofac Orthop (1990), 98:22–28.

INDEX

Note: Page numbers in *italics* refer to illustrations; page numbers followed by t refer to tables.